# Manual of Laboratory Testing Methods for Dental Restorative Materials

# Manual of Laboratory Testing Methods for Dental Restorative Materials

*Dr Paromita Mazumdar and Dr Deepshikha Chowdhury*

WILEY Blackwell

This edition first published 2021


*Registered Offices*
John Wiley & Sons, Inc., 111 River Street, Hoboken, NJ 07030, USA
John Wiley & Sons Ltd, The Atrium, Southern Gate, Chichester, West Sussex, PO19 8SQ, UK

*Editorial Office*
9600 Garsington Road, Oxford, OX4 2DQ, UK

For details of our global editorial offices, customer services, and more information about Wiley products visit us at www.wiley.com.

Wiley also publishes its books in a variety of electronic formats and by print-on-demand. Some content that appears in standard print versions of this book may not be available in other formats.



*Library of Congress Cataloging-in-Publication Data*

Names: Mazumdar, Paromita, author. | Chowdhury, Deepshikha, author.
Title: Manual of laboratory testing methods for dental restorative materials / Dr Paromita Mazumdar, Dr Deepshikha Chowdhury.
Description: First edition. | Hoboken, NJ : Wiley-Blackwell, 2021. | Includes bibliographical references and index.
Identifiers: LCCN 2021015274 (print) | LCCN 2021015275 (ebook) | ISBN 9781119687993 (paperback) | ISBN 9781119688006 (adobe pdf) | ISBN 9781119688020 (epub)
Subjects: MESH: Dental Materials–standards | Dental Restoration, Permanent | Materials Testing | Biofilms
Classification: LCC RK652.5 (print) | LCC RK652.5 (ebook) | NLM WU 190 | DDC 617.6/95–dc23
LC record available at https://lccn.loc.gov/2021015274
LC ebook record available at https://lccn.loc.gov/2021015275

Cover Design: Wiley
Cover Images: © Deepshikha Chowdhury and Paromita Mazumdar

Set in 9.5/12.5pt STIXTwoText by Straive, Pondicherry, India
Printed and bound by CPI Group (UK) Ltd, Croydon, CR0 4YY

C106719_040821

# Contents

# Preface

Throughout our academic life either as a student, or during our role play as a teacher, instructor or supervisor for dissertation or short study designing we always felt that there was a need of a manual describing the methods and techniques for laboratory methods when we embark on a bench study. This manual may be seen as an answer to our thoughts and rigours that we faced.

A number of dental materials are used in the oral cavity for various purpose which includes restorations, endodontic treatment, orthodontic applications, surgical, and prosthodontic treatment.

Many materials used in restorative dentistry are supplied as two or more components which are eventually mixed together and undergo a chemical reaction, during which the various properties may change dramatically. The set material may be a rigid solid or a flexible rubber depending upon the chemical nature of the product. The acceptance of such a product by the dentist depends upon the properties of the unmixed paste, the properties during mixing and setting and the properties of the set material. The properties of the set material can be conveniently divided into the following categories: mechanical properties, thermal properties, chemical properties, biological properties, and other physical properties.

As post graduate trainees, researchers and practitioners, there is a need of evidence-based application of the materials. Post graduate trainees face the difficulty of not having a clear idea about the vastness of the course and the syllabus. Also, a certain amount of time is required to gain a familiarity to the course. A thesis or a dissertation is required to be submitted for the fulfillment of the post graduate masters course and this manual will clearly enumerate the tests done to evaluate the different properties of dental materials like mechanical, physical and optical properties.

The manual consists of seven chapters based on the different properties of dental restorative materials and the mode of testing these properties. A glossary of key terms is provided separately.

Chapter 1 consists of the assessment of various mechanical properties of dental restorative materials that are commonly tested such as tensile strength, diametral compression test, compressive strength, flexural strength, resistance to fatigue, hardness, elastic modulus, fracture toughness and bond strength. Chapter 2 deals with the assessment of various physical properties such as surface roughness, water sorption, viscosity and flow, surface tension and wettability, microleakage, interfacial adaptation, film thickness, and radiopacity. Chapter 3 provides an insight into isolation and identification of oral microflora including both the culture method and the molecular biology techniques. Chapter 4 will give an idea about the assessment of biocompatibility of dental restorative materials which has been segregated based on the testing hierarchy. The different dimensions of color along with the different techniques of assessing colour of restorative materials has been detailed in Chapter 5. Chapter 6 delves into various methods of simulation of the oral environment such as the simulation of saliva, temperature change in the oral cavity, masticatory forces, pH cycling, tooth brushing and periodontium without which translational research will be incomplete. Chapter 7 provides an idea on biofilm in the oral cavity.

For researchers pertaining to dentistry or field of materials, the handbook will provide an insight into the materials used in dentistry, the properties studied, the methods used to study the properties and their respective advantages and disadvantages.

For the clinicians, this handbook will be one of its kind which will help to generate an interest and curiosity about the materials being used in individual practice.

In a nutshell, the manual on testing methods will be a helpful addition to any institute library or personal collection since this aspect of material science has never been explained before. A serious attempt at delving into the minds of young researchers has led to the conceptualization of the manuscript.

We sincerely hope the manual will add value to our intended readers.

***Dr Paromita Mazumdar***
***Dr Deepshikha Chowdhury***

## Acknowledgement

Our special thanks to Dr. Amit Roy Chowdhury, Professor, Aerospace Engineering and Applied Mechanics, Indian Institute of Engineering Science and Technology, Shibpur, West Bengal, India, for his guidance and suggestions.

We are grateful to Dr. Pallab Datta, Assistant Professor, Centre for Healthcare Science and Technology, Indian Institute of Engineering Science and Technology, Shibpur, West Bengal, India, for his priceless and benevolent guidance along with unstained co-operation.

Our sincere thanks to Ms. Preeti Verma, Senior Research Scholar, Department of Botany, Calcutta University, West Bengal, India, for her valuable suggestions, excellent supervision, exceptionally able guidance and constant encouragement.

We are thankful to Ms. Deepanwita Chowdhury, Masters in Life Sciences, Mount Carmel College, Bengaluru, Karnataka, India for her cooperation and encouraging support.

Our heartfelt thanks to Ms. Loan Nguyen, Ms. Anupama Sreekanth and Ms. Tanya McMullin, John Wiley & Sons, United Kingdom for their immense contribution, guidance, suggestions and cooperation throughout the entire process of writing and publishing this manual.

We are grateful to our families, friends and colleagues for their moral support and constant encouragement which has helped us in accomplishing our work.

## Glossary of Key Terms

**Absorption** Absorption of light takes place when matter captures electromagnetic radiation, converting the energy of photons to internal energy.

**Aerobic microbes** microorganisms that can survive and grow in an oxygenated environment.

**Aliquot** A representative sample of a fixed proportion.

**Anerobic microbes** microorganisms that do not require oxygen for growth. It may react negatively or die in the presence of oxygen.

**Assay** the testing of a material to determine its ingredients and quality.

**Biocompatibility** Ability of a material to elicit an appropriate biological response on a given application in the body. It is the quality of not having toxic or injurious effects on biological systems.

**Biofilm** aggregate of microorganisms in which cells that are frequently embedded within a self produced matrix of extracellular polymeric substance adhere to each other and/or to the surface.

**Carcinogenicity** The ability or tendency of a substance to induce tumors (benign or malignant) and increase the malignancy.

**Commensalism** a relationship between two organisms where one benefits but the other is neutral.

**Compressive Strength** Maximum stress a material can sustain under crush loading.

**Compressive Stress** Compressive force per unit area perpendicular to the direction of applied force.

**Contact angle** Angle of intersection between a liquid and a surface of a solid that is measured from the solid surface through the liquid to the liquid/vapor tangent line originating at the terminus of the liquid/solid interface.

**Cyclic loading** Repeated or fluctuating application of forces in structural components.

**Cytotoxicity** the quality of being toxic to cells.

**Degree of conversion** Percentage of carbon–carbon double bonds converted to carbon–carbon single bonds during curing to form a polymeric resin.

**Demineralisation** Loss of minerals from the dental hard tooth tissues.

**Elastic Modulus (also modulus of elasticity and Young's modulus)** Stiffness of a material that is calculated as the ratio of elastic stress to elastic strain.

**Extraction ratio** Ratio of the surface area or mass of the test sample to the volume of the extractant used. It is used in biocompatibility testing of dental materials.

**Flexural strength (bending strength or modulus of rupture)** Force per unit area at the instant of fracture in a test specimen subjected to flexural loading.

**Flexural stress (bending stress)** Force per unit area of a material that is subjected to flexural loading.

**Flow** Relative ability of a wax to plastically deform when it is heated slightly above body temperature.

**Fracture toughness** Ability of a material to absorb elastic energy and to deform plastically before fracturing; measured as the total area under a plot of tensile stress versus strain.

**Genotoxicity** the property of physical or chemical substances that damages the genetic information within a cell causing mutations, which may often lead to cancer.

**Hardness** Hardness is a measure of the resistance to localized plastic deformation induced by either mechanical indentation or abrasion.

**LAB** The 'L' value for each scale indicates the level of light or dark, the 'A' value redness or greenness, and the 'B' value yellowness or blueness. All three values are required to completely describe an object's color.

**Microflora** collective term for all microorganisms.

**Microleakage** The flow of oral fluids and bacteria into the microscopic gap between a prepared tooth surface and a restorative material.

**Mutagenicity** The property which induces mutations in an organism.

**Pathogen** microorganism that causes disease.

**Reflection** Reflection is the change in direction of a wavefront at an interface between two different media so that the wavefront returns into the medium from which it originated.

**Remineralization** Replacement of lost minerals from the dental hard tooth tissues.

**Saturation** saturation is the purity of a color. It is the color of an area judged in proportion to its brightness.

**Sensitivity** ability of a test to correctly identify those with the disease (true positive).

**Shear strength** Shear stress at the point of fracture.

**Shear stress** Ratio of shear force to the original cross-sectional area parallel to the direction of the applied force.

**Specificity** ability of a test to correctly identify those without the disease (true negative).

**Spectral reflectance** The reflectance spectrum or spectral reflectance curve is the plot of the reflectance as a function of wavelength.

**Surface tension** A measurement of the cohesive energy present at an interface.

**Tensile strength (ultimate tensile strength)** Tensile stress at the instant of fracture.

**Tensile stress** Ratio of tensile force to the original cross sectional area perpendicular to the direction of applied force.

**Teratogenicity** capacity of a substance to cause foetal abnormalities when administered during pregnancy.

**Transmission** Transmission of light is the moving of electromagnetic waves (whether visible light, radio waves, ultraviolet, etc.) through a material.

**Toxicity** adverse effects that a chemical or physical agent may produce within a living organism.

**Viscosity** Resistance of a fluid to flow.

## About the Companion Website

The companion website for this book is at

**www.wiley.com/go/mazumdar/dental-restorative-materials**

The website contains –

- All figures from the book as downloadable PowerPoint slides
- A video demonstrating a universal testing machine

Scan this QR code to visit the companion website.

# Introduction

Dental materials are a wide variety of materials which have been used in preventive and restorative dentistry in order to preserve and enhance oral health. Different materials such as ivory, sea shells, ceramic, and metals have been used historically, and some of them are still in use. There is a constant search for a material that fulfills the requirements of an ideal restorative material.

The requirements for an ideal restorative material are as follows:

- Biocompatibility
- Ability to bond to tooth structure and other restorative materials
- Ability to mimic the natural appearance of the tooth
- Has properties similar to dental tissues
- Ability to repair and regenerate damaged tissue

Studying the properties of these materials along with their interaction in the oral environment allows clinicians to predict the clinical performance in the oral cavity.

Several in vitro tests are proposed to evaluate different properties of dental materials, to study the tooth restoration or tooth substitute material and the intervention system. Each test has its design and evaluates specific properties. In order to seek for standardized testing protocols, an international organization was created to act in that direction. The main guidance for dental materials laboratory testing recommended by International Organization for Standardization (ISO) is tabulated as follows.

*Manual of Laboratory Testing Methods for Dental Restorative Materials*, First Edition.
Paromita Mazumdar and Deepshikha Chowdhury.

Companion website: www.wiley.com/go/mazumdar/dental-restorative-materials

**Table 1** ISO specifications to guide dental tests.

| | |
|---|---|
| 1559:1995 | Dental materials – alloys for dental amalgam |
| 1564:1995 | Dental aqueous impression materials based on agar |
| 1942-2:1989 | Dental vocabulary – part 2: dental materials |
| 6876:2001 | Dental root canal sealing materials |
| 7405:1997 | Dentistry – preclinical evaluation of biocompatibility of medical devices used in dentistry test methods for dental materials |
| 7491:2000 | Dental materials – determination of colour stability |
| 9333:1990 | Dentistry – brazing materials |
| 10271:2001 | Dental metallic materials – corrosion test methods |
| 11245:1999 | Dental restorations – phosphate-bonded refractory die materials |
| TS 11405:2003 | Dental materials – testing of adhesion to tooth structure |
| TS 14569-1:1999 | Dental materials – guidance on testing of wear – Part 1: wear by toothbrushing |

The following chapters present the different techniques of testing the dental restorative materials which have been categorized based on the different properties.

# 1

# Assessment of Mechanical Properties of Dental Restorative Materials

**KEY CONCEPTS**

- Knowledge of properties of dental restorative materials.
- Ability to differentiate between each type of mechanical properties.
- Understanding of the type of sample preparation required for the different testing modalities.
- Working principle of the equipment used.
- Different applications of the universal testing machine.

In the oral environment, restorations are subjected to stresses from mastication. These forces act on teeth and/ or material producing different reactions that lead to deformation, which can ultimately compromise their durability over time [1–5].When a specific force or load is applied to a body, a reaction of the same intensity and with opposite direction is produced which causes an internal tension. Hence, it is possible to quantify the reaction that resulted by the applied external load. Since shape and dimensions of specimens under test can be measured, one can calculate stress by the reason between force and unit area.

Depending on the applied load characteristics and consequent stress, different reactions from the tested material may occur. The stress can result in structural alteration of original dimensions. The rate between this alteration by the original dimension results in deformation, that is defined as strain. The stress–strain ratio of a material is relevant to determine its mechanical behavior. For each material, there is a stress–strain proportional relationship, establishing a stress–strain curve. If there is a stress relief during loading and no permanent deformation occurs, it demonstrated its elasticity. This proportion occurs until a limit point that is defined as proportional limit and deformation as elastic deformation. In this point, the maximum stress of a material will withstand without permanent deformation. As stress–strain is proportional until this point, there is a constant proportionality. It determines the elasticity of a material and is calculated by the ratio of stress–strain curve within the elastic limit. This proportionality is defined as modulus of elasticity or Young's modulus. This value will measure the stiffness of such material. However, when the applied load

*Manual of Laboratory Testing Methods for Dental Restorative Materials*, First Edition.
Paromita Mazumdar and Deepshikha Chowdhury.

Companion website: www.wiley.com/go/mazumdar/dental-restorative-materials

exceeds this point, irreversible deformation occurs, resulting in permanent or plastic deformation. Each material presents a resistance to deformation, and after this point, it will result in its rupture. In this point ultimate strength value is obtained. Toughness is the resistance of a material to fracture and corresponds to the amount of energy required to cause it [6]. All these concepts can be applied in clinical situations as many complex forces occur in the oral cavity and tend to deform the material (tensile, compressive, shear, bending forces), the knowledge and interpretation of how these materials behave under such forces are important to understand the performance of the material. Thus the various mechanical parameters that are evaluated for the suitability of a product for any application in the field of conservative dentistry are as follows:

**Good to Know**

The Universal Testing Machine is named so as it is capable of testing compression, tension, bending and flexion.

It works by measuring the stress–strain relationship of each material.

Tensile strength, diametral compression test, compressive strength, flexural strength, resistance to fatigue, hardness, elastic modulus, fracture toughness and bond strength.

Different equipment are used for testing different mechanical properties. Each of these tests may be conducted using either tooth or materials or both (in case of bonded structures). All these tests require variations in the assembly. Most of the tests except hardness require the use of Universal Testing Machine (UTM) where the sample preparations differ for each test. For instance, if tensile testing is done on a sample, the shape of the sample is dumb bell shaped; it is designed so that the specimen can be gripped at each end and stretched. For compressive strength testing, cylindrical-shaped specimens are tested. Bar-shaped specimens are used for flexural strength testing (as shown in Figures 1.1 and 1.2).

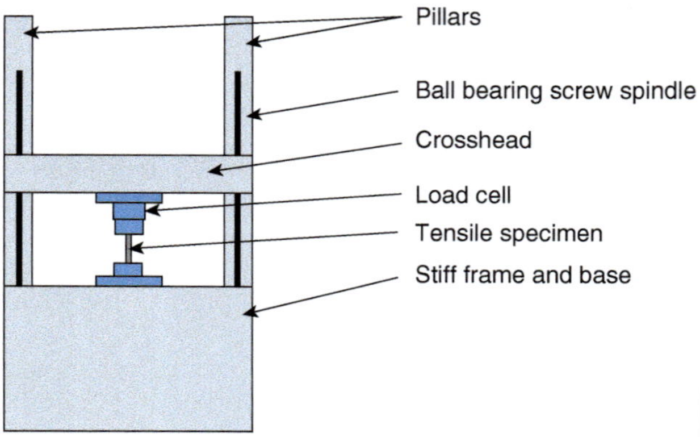


**Figure 1.1** Universal testing machine.

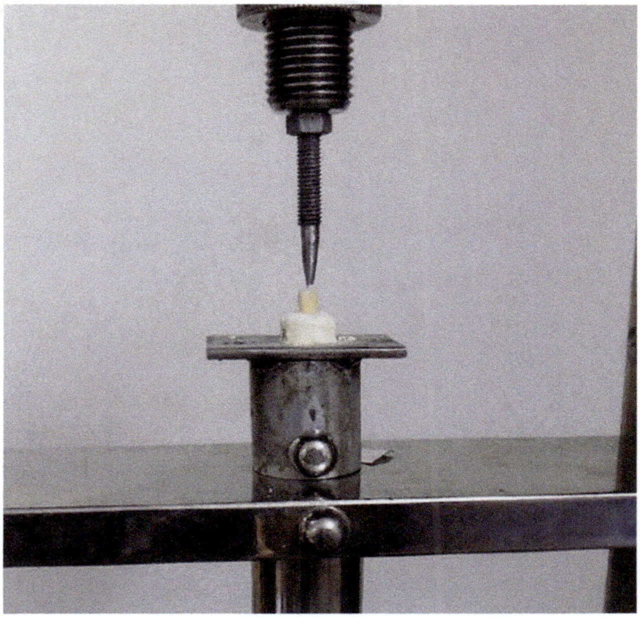

**Figure 1.2** Tooth sample testing.

## 1.1 Tensile Strength

When a body is subjected to axial forces in a straight line and in opposite directions, it results in tension. The resistance of the material to this load is called tensile strength. The length alteration that results from the application of a tensile force on a body before its rupture is defined as elongation. Nominal value of tensile strength is determined by the equation of load and cross-sectional area (Kgf/cm$^2$). Values of stress–strain determine a curve, characterizing the performance of the material under tensile test. From this curve, elastic modulus, ultimate tensile strength, resilience and toughness of such product can be registered [7]. Tensile testing is normally applied to materials which are placed under loading that is generally applied in different directions, as the opposing cusps move over the restoration surface. Loads that stretch or elongate a material cause tensile stresses (as shown in Figures 1.3–1.5).

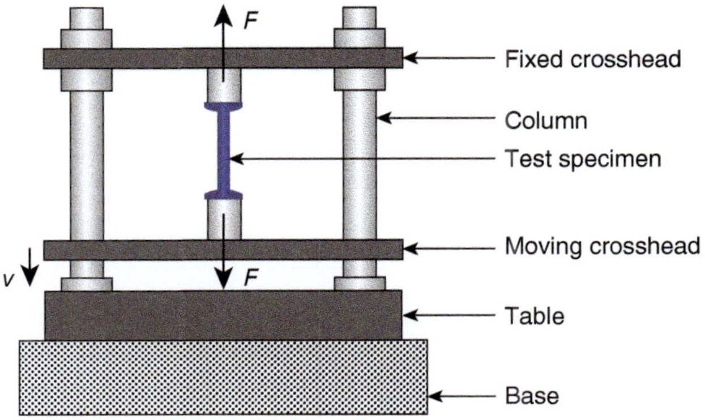


**Figure 1.3** Tensile strength assessment.

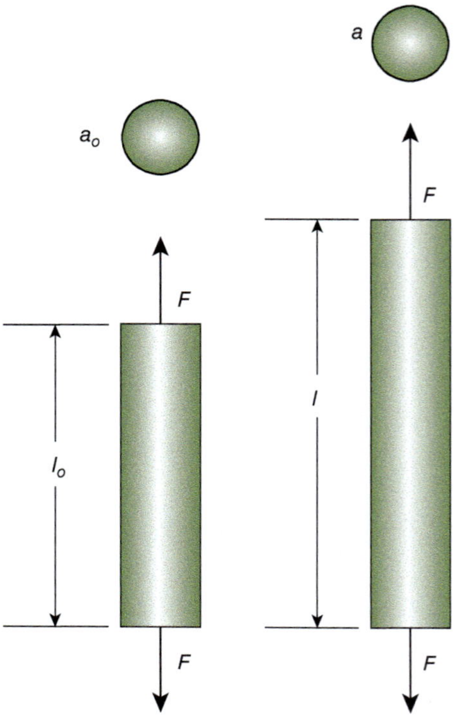


**Figure 1.4** Tensile strength assessment.

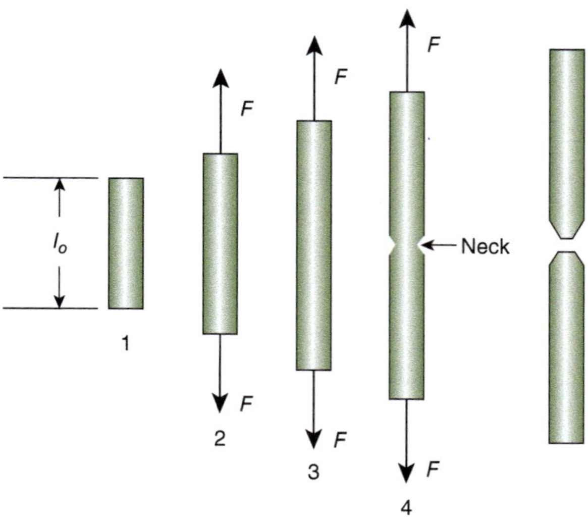


**Figure 1.5** 1, No load; 2, uniform elongation; 3, maximum load; 4, necking.

| Good to Know |
| --- |
| For a DTS test, the fracture line doesn't always occur along the central line, thus giving false results and making the test inaccurate. |

The diametral tensile strength (DTS) test is useful for materials that exhibit very limited plastic deformation and where information regarding stretching or elongation resistance is required. The DTS is a property described by American Dental Association (ADA)/American National Standards Institute (ANSI) Specification 27 for characterizing dental composite restoratives (DCR). It represents the minimal stress that a body will withstand without rupture when tensile loads are applied. The DTS test is considered useful because masticatory forces are frequently applied obliquely and tend to create tensile stress. A UTM is generally used to determine the tensile strength of a material. Materials which plastically deform would produce erroneous DTS values and also would be expected to display strain rate sensitivity. Composite resins are subjected to complex intraoral forces during mastication and parafunctional habits. Of the three tests used in this study to replicate intraoral forces, diametral tensile is the most difficult to interpret. Failure must occur in the center of the specimen along the diameter due to tensile forces if the diametral test is to yield useful results. The method was used to evaluate the influence of different cross-head speeds on DTS of a resin composite material (Tetric N-Ceram) by Anubhav Sood et al. in 2015 where they found that the cross-head speed variations did not have a significant effect on the DTS of the resin composite [8].

## 1.2 Diametral Compression Test

Rupture under low tension characterizes fragile materials, susceptible to brittleness. In these cases, tensile strength is not indicated to evaluate material reaction, because of the low cohesive condition. An alternative method of tensile strength is calculated by compressive testing. It is a relatively simple and reproducible test. It is defined as diametral compression test for tension or indirect tension. Disk sample is necessary to conduct this test, where it is compressed diametrically introducing tensile stress in the material in the plane of the force application by the test. This is calculated by the formula: $2P/\pi \times D \times T$, where: $P$ = load applied, $D$ = diameter of the disk, $T$ = thickness of the disk, $\pi$ = constant [9, 10] (as shown in Figure 1.6).

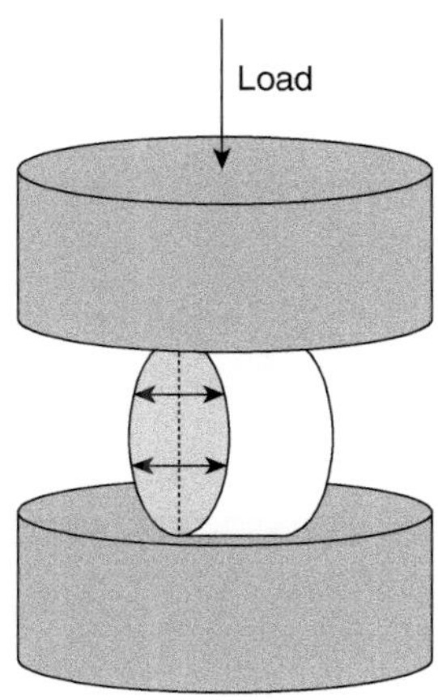


**Figure 1.6** Diametral compressive strength assessment. *Source:* Cefaly [9], Cattani-Lorente [10].

## 1.3 Compressive Strength

Compressive testing is normally applied to materials that are expected to be placed in situations of occlusal loading. Since most of mastication forces are compressive in nature, it is important to investigate materials under this condition. To test compressive strength of a material, two axial sets of force are applied to a sample in an opposite direction, in order to approximate the molecular structure of the material. Here, cylindrical-shaped specimens are tested. The dimensions of the samples should have a relation of length to diameter of 2:1. When this proportion is exceeded, it can

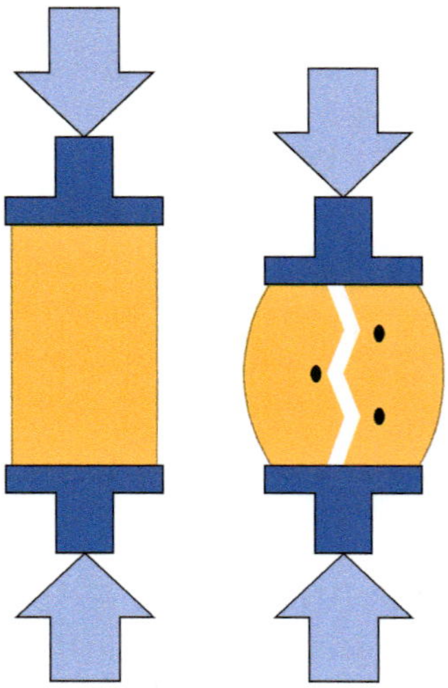

Figure 1.7 Direction of force is perpendicular to the object.

result in undesirable bending of the specimen. In the same manner of tensile strength, nominal value of compressive strength also is determined by the reason of load by cross-sectional area (Kgf/cm$^2$). Stress–strain curve of investigated material is determined in the same manner as established to tensile tests. Thus, the elastic modulus can also be determined by the stress–strain ratio in the elastic region [11] (as shown in Figures 1.7 and 1.8).

## 1.4 Flexural Strength

The flexural strength of a material is its ability to bend before it breaks. It is obtained when the ultimate flexibility of one material is achieved before its proportional limit. This is a measure of the strength of a beam of restorative material supported at each end and subjected to a static load. Stresses on the upper surface of the beam tend to be compressive, whilst those on the lower surface are tensile. This test may be considered to combine elements of tensile and compressive testing. Flexural forces are the result of forces generated in clinical situations and the dental materials need to withstand repeated flexing, bending, and twisting. A high flexural strength is desired once these materials are under the action of chewing stress that might induce permanent deformation. To evaluate flexural strength of a dental material, bar-shaped specimens with dimension of 25 mm in length,2 mm in width and 2 mm in height (ISO 9917 – 212) are generally used. Specimens are placed on two supports and a load is applied at the center. This test is known as three-point bending test. The load at yield is the sample material's flexural strength that is calculated by the following formula:

$$3Pl/2bd^2 \tag{1.1}$$

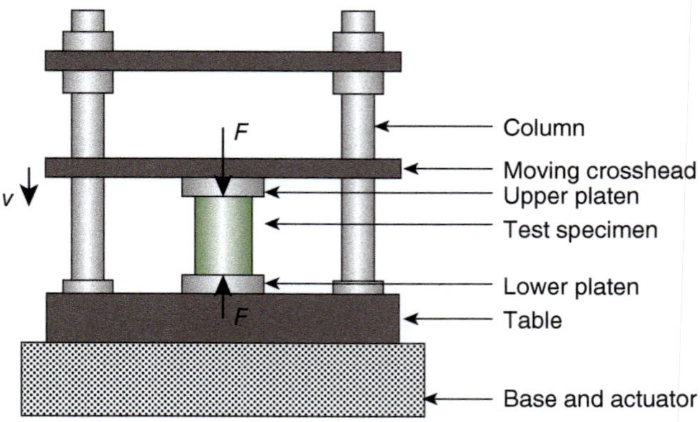


Figure 1.8 Schematic representation of the set-up for compressive strength.

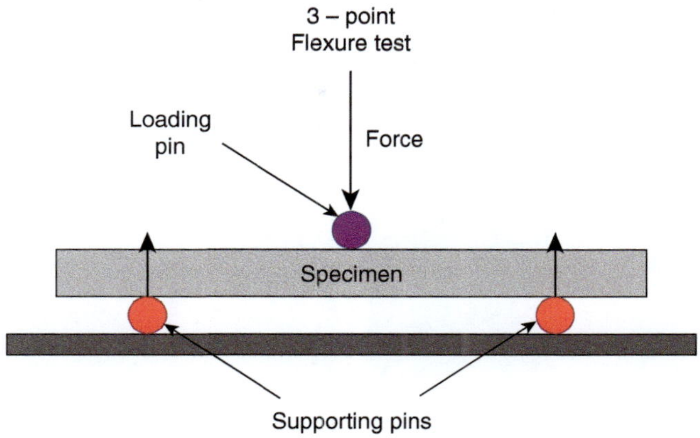


**Figure 1.9** Schematic representation of flexural strength assessment. *Source:* Anusavice [12], Anusavice [13], International Organization for standardization [14].

where $P$ is the ultimate load at fracture, $l$ is the distance of the supports, $b$ is the width of the specimen, and $d$ is the thickness of the specimen [12–14] (as shown in Figure 1.9).

| Good to Know |
|---|
| Apart from the three-point bending test, there are four-point bending tests and biaxial bending tests. |

The four-point flexure test also employ specimens that are loaded symmetrically at two locations with loading rollers, and the distance between loading points is usually one-third or one-fourth of the support span length. In four-point flexure test, maximum bending occurs between the loading points, whereas in three-point flexure test, the maximum bending occurs below the loading roller.

Bi-axial flexure testing is a commonly used technique for the evaluation of dental ceramics. Here force is given in two axes. Bi-axial flexure testing is independent of specimen geometry and force direction

## 1.5 Resistance to Fatigue

The behaviour of materials under the action of low but intermittent stresses shows the resistance to fatigue. This method permits measurement of a fatigue limit, with no fracture, at a given number of stress cycles. Compressive fatigue curves are generated when different materials are submitted to cyclic compressive stress. Tests are made with the test machine operation at a given loading frequency. The presence of defects in the microstructure of the restoration or specimen submitted to high or low stresses leads to the development of cracks. As clinical environment influences are critical factors due to the relatively low stress, these cracks will turn into fracture of the material [12] (as shown in Figures 1.10 and 1.11).

(a) (b)

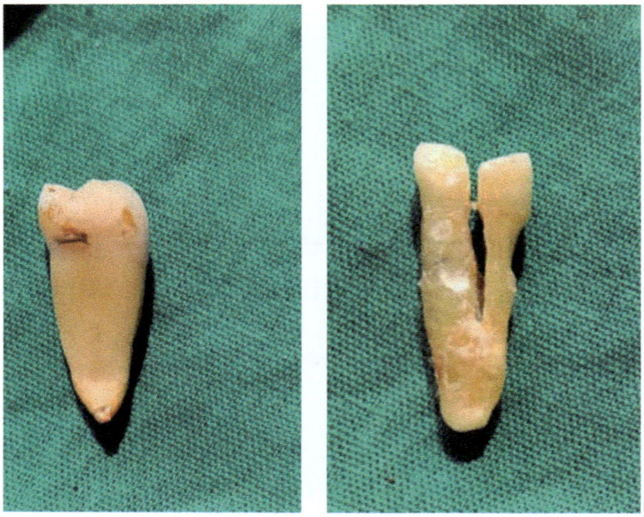

**Figure 1.10** (a) Tooth sample, (b) crack propagation.

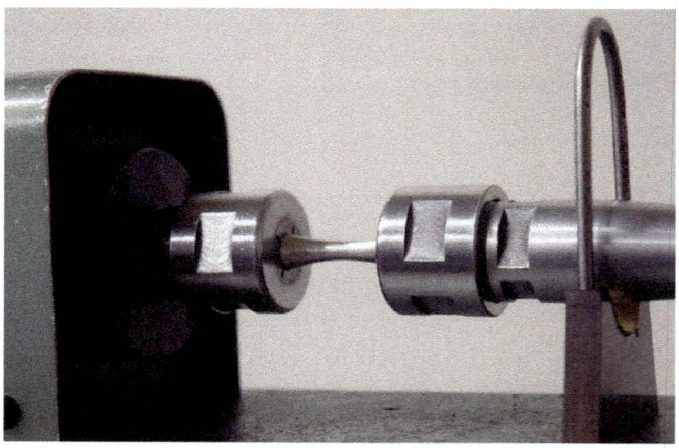

**Figure 1.11** Assessment of resistance to fatigue by cyclic compression stress.

## 1.6 Hardness

Major laboratory tests are performed to investigate products based on their bulk features. Hardness is not an intrinsic material property dictated by precise definitions in terms of fundamental units of mass, length and time. A hardness property value is the result of a defined measurement procedure. The hardness of a material gives an indication of the resistance to penetration when indented by a hard asperity. The value of hardness, often referred to as the hardness number, depends on the method used for its evaluation. Generally, low values of hardness number indicate a soft material and vice versa.

Hardness measurement can be defined as macro or micro, according to the forces applied and displacements obtained. Macro means large, therefore macro hardness is a measurement of the hardness of a material when a large force of greater than 50 N is applied. Macro hardness can be regular or superficial. In regular macro hardness, it is applicable to large area with deep penetration, whereas in superficial macro hardness, it is applicable to large area with shallow penetration. Macro hardness tests can be applied with heavier loads than micro indentation tests.

Micro hardness is a broadly used term referring to the testing of hardness involving materials by using small applied loads. A more appropriate term to describe this is micro indentation hardness testing. In this testing method, the use of a diamond indenter with a particular shape is used to make an impression called a "test load" or "applied force", which can be at 1–1000 gf, on the material under testing. Normally, micro indentation tests involve 2 N forces, which are roughly equivalent to 200 gf. This force can produce an indentation of around 50 μm. Because of its specificity, this type of testing is applicable in cases where there is a need to watch for hardness changes on a microscopic level.

Rockwell, Brinell and Vickers hardness tests are applied for macro hardness testing, whereas Knoop hardness and Vickers hardness tests are done for microhardness testing.

Macro hardness testing has industrial applications such as testing hardness of steel, aluminium. Micro hardness test is applicable in dentistry for assessment of tooth samples and dental materials such as metals, ceramics and composites. Micro hardness tests are useful in giving required data when taking measurements of single microstructures situated within a bigger matrix and testing foil-like or thin materials.

The usual method to achieve hardness value is to measure the depth or area of an indentation left by an indenter of a specific shape with a specific force applied for a specific time.

Vickers and Knoop both involve the use of diamond pyramid indenters. In the case of Vickers hardness, the diamond pyramid has a square base, whilst for Knoop hardness, one axis of the diamond pyramid is much larger than the other.

The Vickers hardness test method consists of indenting the test material with a diamond indenter, in the form of a right pyramid with a square base and an angle of 136° between opposite faces subjected to a load of 1–100 Kgf. The load is normally applied for 10–15 seconds. The two diagonals of the indentation left in the surface of the material after removal of the load are measured using a microscope and their average is calculated. The area of the sloping surface of the indentation is calculated. It is suitable to be applied to determine the hardness of small areas and for very hard materials.

Knoop hardness is more sensitive to surface characteristics of the material. The Knoop indenter is a diamond ground to pyramidal form that produces a diamond-shaped indentation having approximate ratio between long and short diagonals of 7 : 1. The depth of indentation is about 1/30 of its length. When measuring the Knoop hardness, only the longest diagonal of the indentation is measured, and this is used in the following formula with the load used to calculate Knoop Hardness Number (KHN). Knoop hardness test is applied to evaluate enamel and dentine structures. One of the major difficulties is the requirement of a high polished flat surface that is more time-consuming and more care taking compared to other tests.

Comparing the indentations made with Knoop and Vickers Diamond Pyramid indenters for a given load and test material, there are some technical differences as follows:

- Vickers indenter penetrates about twice as deep as Knoop indenter.
- Vickers indentation diagonal is about 1/3 of the length of Knoop major diagonal.

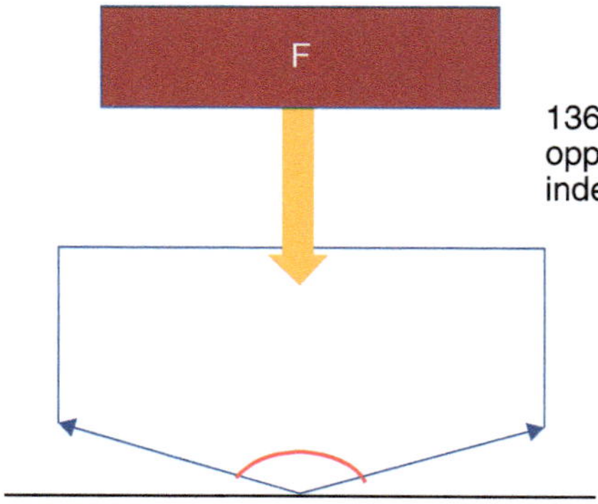


**Figure 1.12** Vickers hardness testing.

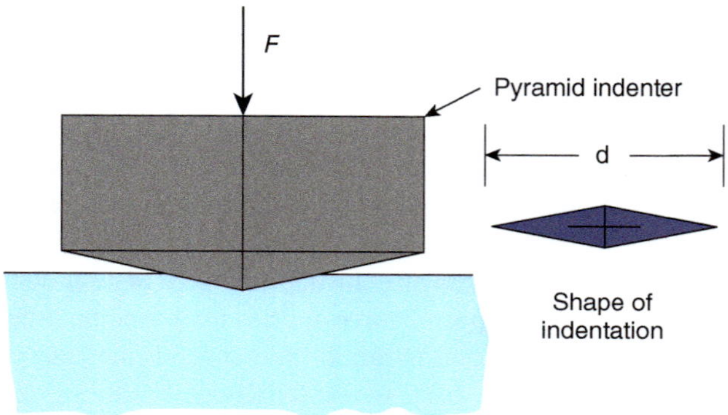


**Figure 1.13** Knoop hardness testing.

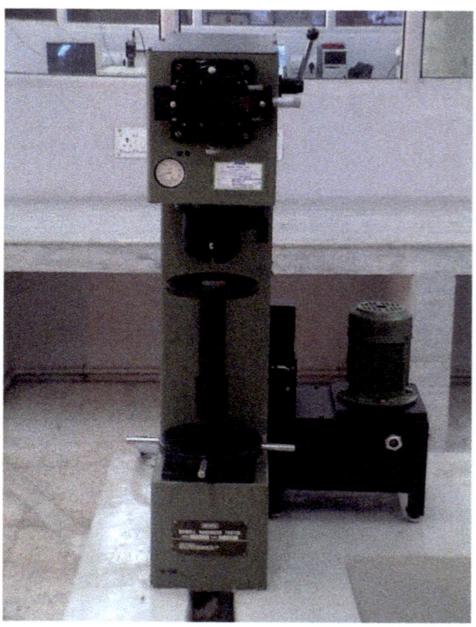

**Figure 1.14** Vickers hardness tester.

- Vickers test is less sensitive to surface conditions than Knoop test.
- Vickers test is more sensitive to measurement errors than Knoop test.
- Vickers test is best for small rounded areas, whereas Knoop test is best for small elongated areas (as shown in Figures 1.12–1.14).

The Brinell hardness test method consists of indenting the material with a 10 mm diameter hardened steel or carbide ball subjected to a load. It is the oldest method to measure surface hardness and is applicable to test metals and alloys (as shown in Figure 1.15).

Measurements are normally made using a microscope since the indentations are often too small to be seen with the naked eye. The hardness is a function of the diameter of the circle for Brinell

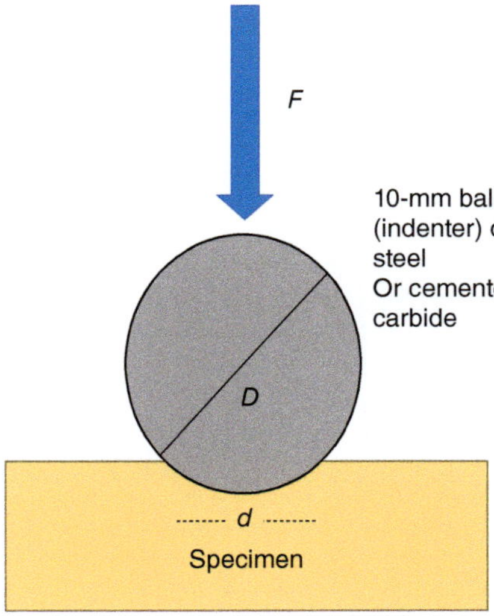


Figure 1.15 Brinell hardness testing.

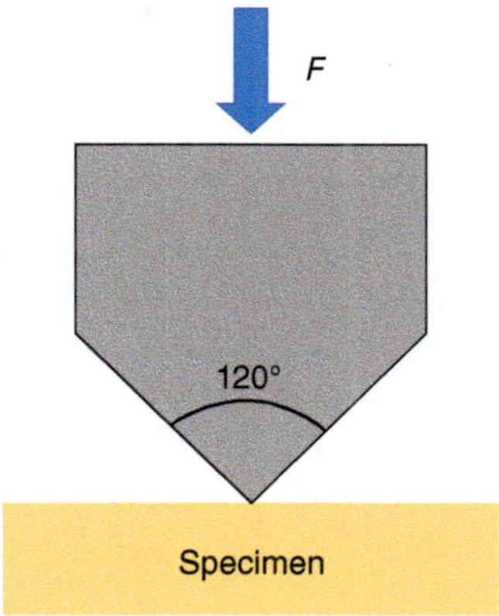


Figure 1.16 Rockwell hardness testing. *Source:* Vieira [4]. Licensed under CC BY 4.0.

hardness and the distance across the diagonal axes for Vickers and Knoop hardness. Allowance is naturally made for the magnitude of the applied loads. In the case of Rockwell hardness, a direct measurement of the depth of penetration of a conical diamond indenter is made. The Rockwell hardness test method consists of indenting the test material with a diamond cone or hardened steel ball indenter. This method is useful to evaluate surface hardness of plastic materials used in dentistry [4] (as shown in Figure 1.16).

**Good to Know**

All materials require different hardness testing. The specificity of a hardness tester is dependent on the following factors:

a) Material of the indenter
b) Shape and size of the indenter and the sample to be tested.
c) Loading parameter (amount of force it can apply)

Hardness tests are extremely used and have important applicability on Dentistry. Hardness test can evaluate the degree of mineralization of a dental substrate for example. A specific force applied for a specific time and distance provides important data in studies assessing the ability of enamel and dentin remineralization after different treatments as happens in unbalanced situations of des-remineralization. Another important use of this test is to evaluate the degree of polymerization of resin composite and resin cements.

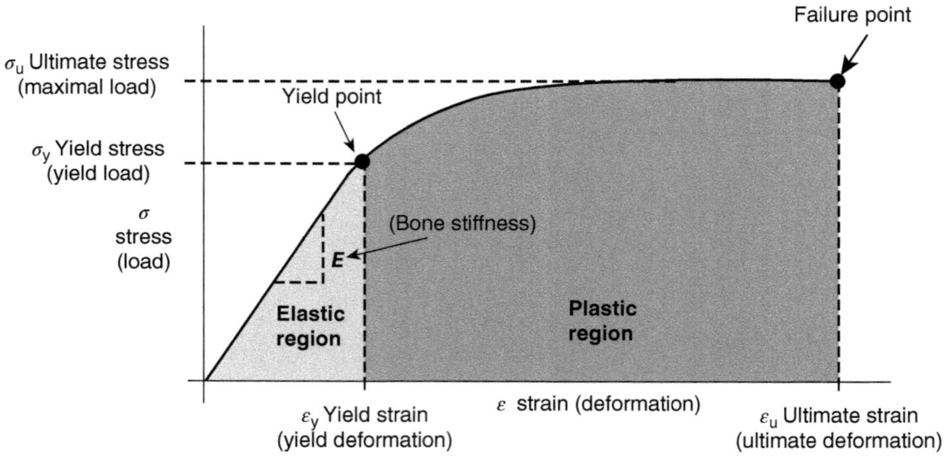


**Figure 1.17** Stress–strain curve for assessment of Young's modulus.

## 1.7 Elastic Modulus

The modulus of elasticity, or measure of a material's stiffness, is also important in relation to anticipated longevity of a restoration. An elastic material (one with a low elastic modulus) will deform when a load is placed on it but will return to its original shape once the load falls below the elastic limit of the material. As a general rule, restorative materials need to be very stiff (high elastic modulus), so that under load the elastic deformation will be very small. An exception to this is in the Class V situation. Micro-filled composite materials have a lower modulus of elasticity than hybrid composite materials; this may be why micro-filled materials show higher retention rates in Class V cavities, given that they deform more readily as the tooth deforms at the cervical area under occlusal loading.

Models involving the use of springs and dashpots can be used to explain the elastic and viscoelastic behaviour of materials. When a spring, which represents an elastic material, is fixed at one end and a load applied at the other, it becomes instantaneously extended. When the load is removed, it immediately recovers its original length. This behaviour is analogous to that of a perfectly elastic material. The two things that characterize the material are firstly the perfect recovery after removal of the force and secondly the lack of any time dependency of either the deformation under load or the recovery after removal of the applied force. The extent of deformation under load is characterized by the modulus of elasticity of the material (analogous to the spring constant of the spring) (as shown in Figure 1.17).

## 1.8 Fracture Toughness

Fracture toughness determines the resistance of a material to the propagation of a crack. This test has been considered to be efficient given that other parameters can be derived from it. It should be kept in mind, however, that fracture toughness measures the failure of a material after one continuous period of loading, whereas fatigue strength experiments measure crack propagation after repeated applications of a small cyclic load. A UTM (Instron) is used to apply a central load to the specimen in a three-point bending mode at a cross-head speed of 0.125 mm/minute. Fracture of the specimen is identified by a sudden drop in load during the test. Visual examination of the fractured parts is performed to ensure that the fracture plane is through the notch, and that it is perpendicular to the vertical and horizontal planes through the center of the specimens.

The fracture toughness was then calculated by:

$$\text{Kic} = \left(PL / bw1.5\right) f\left(a / w\right) \tag{1.2}$$

The variables are defined as: Kic is the stress intensity factor, *P* is the load at fracture, *L* is the span, distance between the supports, *w* is the width of the specimen, *b* is the thickness of the specimen, and *a* is the crack length.

| **Good to Know** |
|---|
| Cross-head speed is also known as deformation rate. It is measured in mm/min. Every material has different average cross-head speeds recommended by ISO 4049. For e.g. resin-based composites have a speed of (0.75 ± 0.25 mm/min). |

## 1.9 Nanoindentation

With nanoscience gaining popularity, nanoindenters have advantages over traditional mechanical testing by providing both elastic modulus and hardness data of the tested samples. Nanoindentation is conducted with a calibrated Berkovich diamond indenter tip. A Berkovich tip is a three-sided pyramidal indenter.

During the nanoindentation process, a calibrated indenter tip approaches the surface of the sample. The force–displacement data is used to determine the point of contact. After the sample is contacted, the force is linearly increased and the tip indents into the surface of the sample. A short dwell time occurs at the maximum force and then the sample is unloaded. At the initial point of unloading, the stiffness is measured.

## 1.10 Bond Strength

Longevity of a restoration is predicted to some extent by its adhesive ability, and this in turn can be measured by bond strength testing. An ideal bond strength test should be accurate, clinically reliable and less technique-sensitive. It should involve the use of relatively unsophisticated and inexpensive test protocols. Static tests are categorized into macro-tests where the bond area is $>3\,\text{mm}^2$ and micro-tests with $<3\,\text{mm}^2$ bond area [15].

### 1.10.1 Macro-Test Methods

The macro-bond strength can be measured in shear, tensile or using a push-out protocol.

#### 1.10.1.1 Macro-Shear (SBS) Test

In a shear bond test, two materials are connected via an adhesive agent and loaded in shear until fracture occurs.

#### 1.10.1.2 Macro-Tensile (TBS) Test

In a tensile bond test, load will be exerted on either sides of the test specimen. The specimen can be held by active or passive gripping methods. Active gripping method involves mechanical fastening of specimen to gripping device, such as glue or clamps, whereas in passive gripping method, specimen is placed in a testing device without the aid of glue or mechanical gripping. It can be used to measure, for instance, the bond strength of cements to hard materials such as ceramics and metal alloys [16].

#### 1.10.1.3 Push-Out (PO) Test

In this method, load is applied through a plunger mounted in the UTM. The plunger must provide near-complete coverage of the testing material without touching the substrate. This method is useful to test adhesion of root canal sealers and retention of posts luted in root canals [17].

### 1.10.2 Micro-Test Methods

#### 1.10.2.1 Micro Shear Test

Shear bond strength (SBS) testing with bonded cross-sectional areas of 3 $mm^2$ or less is referred to as "micro" SBS. It permits efficient screening of adhesive systems, regional and depth profiling of a variety of substrates and conservation of teeth. Micro-shear tests remain an extremely useful test for those substrates with properties such as glass ionomers or enamel that make them particularly susceptible to the specimen preparation effects and testing conditions of μTBS testing [18].

#### 1.10.2.2 Micro Tensile Test

Micro-tensile bond test (μTBS) allowed additional research designs that the "macro" tests did not, such as the elimination of tooth dependency through balanced designs. However, there is a difficulty in measuring bond strengths lower than 5 MPa [19].

#### 1.10.2.3 Micro Push-Out Bond Strength

Micro-push-out test is a modification of push-out test where the specimen thickness is less than or equal to 1 $mm^2$ [15].

**Key Points**

1) Tensile strength, diametral compression test, compressive strength, flexural strength, resistance to fatigue, hardness, elastic modulus, fracture toughness are the various mechanical properties that are measured in the field of dental material sciences.
2) Universal Testing Machine (UTM) is used for most of the tests with the only difference being that the sample preparations differ for each test. Hardness testing depends upon the material to be tested.

3) The samples are prepared as per ISO standards to get optimum results. Also, the area which is subjected to the force differs due to the size of the stick/blade.
4) Axial forces in a straight line and in opposite directions result in tension in the body of a material, and the resistance of the material to this load is called tensile strength. Nominal value of tensile strength is determined by the equation of load and cross-sectional area (Kgf/cm$^2$).
5) The diametral tensile strength (DTS) test is useful for materials where information regarding stretching or elongation resistance is required and the failure has to occur along the center of the specimen.
6) Compressive strength is used to test materials which are subjected to occlusally directed forces in the oral cavity.
7) Flexural forces are the forces that generate repeated flexing, bending and twisting of the materials.
8) Resistance to fatigue is the measurement of a fatigue limit, with no fracture, at a given number stress cycles.
9) Hardness of a material gives an indication of the resistance to penetration when indented by a hard asperity.
10) Types of hardness: macro hardness and micro hardness.
11) Macro hardness has force application greater than 50 N, and micro hardness has force application less than 10 N. Macro hardness test is done using Vickers, Rockwell and Brinell hardness tester, whereas micro hardness test is done using Vickers and Knoop hardness tester.

## References


**1** Albers, H.F. (1996). *Tooth-Colored Restoratives*, 8e. Santa Rosa: Alto Books.

**2** Craig, R.G. (1997). *Mechanical Properties. Restorative Dental Materials*, 10e, 56–103. St. Louis: Mosby.

**3** Craig, R.G. (1997). *Optical, Thermal, and Electrical Properties. Restorative Dental Materials*, 10e, 30–55. St. Louis: Mosby.

**4** Vieira, D.F. (1965). *Propriedades mecânicas. Propriedades dos materiais odontológicos*, 31–89. São Paulo, Universidade de São Paulo.

**5** Vieira, D.F. (1965). *Propriedades ou constantes físicas. Propriedades dos materiais odontológicos*, 92–105. São Paulo: Universidade de São Paulo.

**6** Wang, L., Henrique, P., Gonzaga, L., and Carlos, J. (2003). Mechanical properties of dental restorative materials: relative contribution of laboratory tests. *J. Appl. Oral Sci.* 11 (3): 162–167.

**7** Darvell, B.W. (2000). *Mechanical testing. Materials science for Denstistry*, 6e, 1–34. Hong Kong: University of Hong Kong.

**8** Sood, A., Ramarao, S., and Carounanidy, U. (2015). Influence of different crosshead speeds on diametral tensile strength of a methacrylate based resin composite: An in-vitro study. *J. Conserv. Dent.* 18: 214. https://doi.org/10.4103/0972-0707.

**9** Cefaly, D.F.G., Franco, E.B., Mondelli, R.F.L. et al. (2003). Resistência à tração diametral e sorção de água de cimentos de ionômero de vidro usados no Tratamento Restaurador Atraumático. *J. Appl. Oral Sci.* 11 (2): 96–101. https://doi.org/10.1590/S1678-77572003000200003.

**10** Cattani-Lorente, M.A. (1999). Comparative study of the physical properties of a polyacid-modified composite resin and a resin-modified glass ionomer cement. *Dent. Mater.* 15: 21–32.
**11** International Organization for Standardization (1993). *Technical report ISO 9917.* Switzerland: Dental water-based cements.
**12** Anusavice, K.J. (1993). Recent developments in restorative dental ceramics. *J. Am. Dent. Assoc.* 24: 73–84.
**13** Anusavice, K.J. (1983). *Propriedades mecânicas dos materiais dentários. Phillips materiais dentários*, 10e, 28–43. Rio de Janeiro: Guanabara Koogan.
**14** International Organization for standardization (1998). *Technical report ISO 9917-2 Dental water-based cements- Part 2.* Switzerland: Light-activated cements.
**15** Castellan, C.S., Santos-Filho, P.C., Soares, P.V. et al. (2010). Measuring bond strength between fiber post and root dentin: a comparison of different tests. *J. Adhes. Dent.* 12: 477–485.
**16** De Munck, J., Mine, A., Poitevin, A. et al. (2010). Testing bond strength. A review of the literature. *Dent. Mater.* 26: e139–e140.
**17** Jainaen, A., Palamara, J.E., and Messer, H.H. (2007). Push-out bond strengths of the dentine – sealer interface with and without a main cone. *Int. Endod. J.* 40: 882–890.
**18** Armstrong, S., Geraldeli, S., Maia, R. et al. (2010). Adhesion to tooth structure: a critical review of "micro" bond strength test methods. *Dent. Mater.* 26: e50–e62.
**19** Pashley, D.H., Carvalho, R.M., Sano, H. et al. (1999). The microtensile bond test: a review. *J. Adhes. Dent.* 1: 299–309.

# 2

# Assessment of Physical Properties of Dental Restorative Materials

**KEY CONCEPTS**

- In-depth knowledge of the assessment of surface roughness, water sorption, viscosity and flow, surface tension and wettability, microleakage, interfacial adaptation, film thickness, and radiopacity.
- The type of samples which can be tested for each property.
- Working principle of each equipment.

A material's physical properties denote the physical state of materials that are exclusive of their chemical or mechanical components. Some of the common physical properties of dental restorative materials that are commonly explored are surface roughness, water sorption, viscosity and flow, surface tension and wettability, microleakage, interfacial adaptation, film thickness, and radiopacity.

## 2.1 Assessment of Surface Roughness

A solid surface, or more exactly a solid–gas or solid–liquid interface, has a complex structure and complex properties depending on the nature of the solids, the method of surface preparation and the interaction between the surface and the environment. Properties of solid surfaces are crucial to surface interaction because surface properties affect real area of contact, friction, wear and lubrication [1]. According to Phillips, surface roughness is defined as relatively finely spaced surface imperfections whose height, width, and direction establish the predominant surface pattern [2].

As the surface roughness of the restoration increases, the degree of light reflection increases and, consequently, there is a reduction in shine of the restoration. The clinical importance of surface roughness includes its direct effects on plaque accumulation predisposing to secondary caries, wear and an increase in staining susceptibility for tooth-colored restorative materials.

*Manual of Laboratory Testing Methods for Dental Restorative Materials*, First Edition.
Paromita Mazumdar and Deepshikha Chowdhury.

Companion website: www.wiley.com/go/mazumdar/dental-restorative-materials

Surface roughness of a restoration is associated with its inherent characteristics, such as the composition along with the material's exposure, tooth brushing abrasion, low pH food, drinks, and mouth rinse solutions [3].

Various instruments are available for the roughness measurement. The measurement technique can be divided into two broad categories: (i) contact type in which during measurement, a component of the measurement instrument contacts the surface to be measured; and (ii) noncontact type.

A contact-type instrument may damage surfaces when used with a sharp stylus tip, particularly soft surfaces. For these measurements, the normal loads must be low enough so that the contact stresses do not exceed the hardness of the surface to be measured.

The first practical stylus instruments were developed by Abbott and Firestone [1] and Thomas [4]. In 1939, Rank Taylor Hobson in Leicester, England, introduced the first commercial instrument called Talysurf. In 1983, a noncontact optical profiler based on the principle of two-beam optical interferometry was developed and is now widely used in the electronics and optical industries to measure smooth surfaces. In 1985, an atomic force microscope was developed which is basically a nanoprofiler operating at ultra-low loads. It can be used to measure surface roughness with lateral resolution ranging from microscopic to atomic scales. This instrument is commonly used in research to measure roughness with extremely high lateral resolution, particularly nanoscale roughness. The different techniques will be divided into six categories based on the physical principle involved: mechanical stylus method, optical methods, scanning probe microscopy (SPM) methods, fluid methods, electrical method, and electron microscopy methods [5].

### 2.1.1 Mechanical Stylus Method

This method uses an instrument that amplifies and records the vertical motions of a stylus displaced at a constant speed by the surface to be measured. The stylus is mechanically coupled mostly to a linear variable differential transformer (LVDT), an optical or a capacitance sensor. The stylus arm is loaded against the sample, and either the stylus is scanned across the stationary sample surface using a traverse unit at a constant speed or the sample is transported across an optical flat reference. As the stylus or sample moves, the stylus rides over the sample surface detecting surface deviations by the transducer. It produces an analog signal corresponding to the vertical stylus movement. This signal is then amplified, conditioned, and digitized. In order to track the stylus across the surface, force is applied to the stylus. The ability to accurately apply and control this force is critical to the profiler performance. The measurement head uses a wire coil to set a programmable stylus load as low as 0.05 mg. Attached above the stylus flexure pivot is an arm with a magnet mounted to the end. The magnet is held in close proximity to the wire coil, and the coil, when energized, produces a magnetic field that moves the magnet arm. This applied force pushes the stylus arm past its null position to a calibrated force displacement, where the horizontal position of the stylus arm represents zero applied force to the stylus. The force coil mechanism and a sophisticated digital signal processor are used to maintain a constant applied force to the stylus. Styli are made of diamond. The shapes can vary from one manufacturer to another. Chisel-point styli with tips (e.g., $0.25 \times 2.5\,\mu m$) may be used for detection of bumps or other special applications [4].

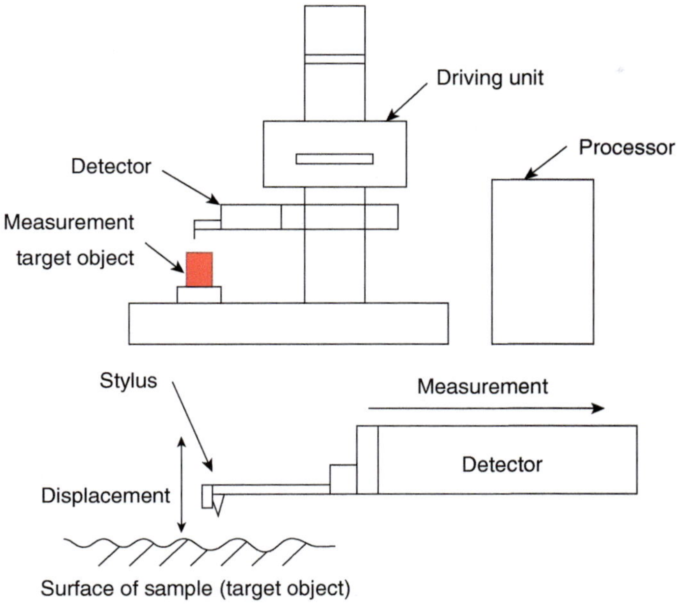


**Figure 2.1** Contact type surface roughness measurement device. *Source:* Thomas [4] and Anonymous [5, 6].

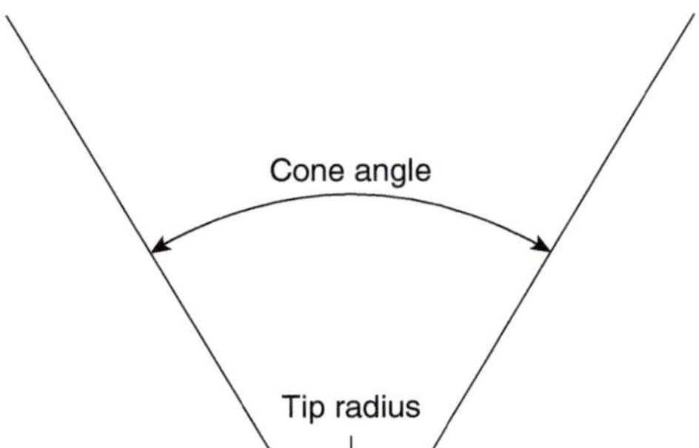


**Figure 2.2** Tip of the stylus. *Source:* Thomas [4] and Anonymous [5, 6].

Conical tips are almost exclusively used for microroughness measurements. According to the international standard (ISO 3274–1975), a stylus is a cone of a 60° to 90° included angle and a (spherical) tip radius of curvature of 2, 5, or 10 μm. The radius of a stylus ranges typically from 0.1 to 0.2 to 25 μm [4–6] (as shown in Figures 2.1 and 2.2).

### 2.1.2 Optical Method

Numerous optical methods have been reported in the literature for measurement of surface roughness. Optical microscopy has been used for overall surveying, which only provides qualitative information. Optical methods may be divided into geometrical and physical methods [4]. Geometrical methods include taper sectioning and light sectioning methods. Physical methods include specular and diffuse reflections, speckle pattern, and optical interference.

#### 2.1.2.1 Taper-Sectioning Method

In this technique, a section is cut through the surface to be examined at a shallow angle θ, thus effectively magnifying height variations by a factor cot $\theta$ and is subsequently examined by an optical microscope. The surface to be sectioned has to be supported with an adherent coating that will prevent smearing of the contour during the sectioning operation. This coating must firmly adhere to the surface, must have a similar hardness, and should not diffuse into the surface. 0.5-mm-thick specimen surfaces need to be used. The specimen is then ground on a surface grinder at a typical taper angle between 1° and 6°. The taper section so produced is lapped, polished, and possibly lightly etched or heat tinted to provide good contrast for the optical examination. The disadvantages of this technique include destruction of the test surface, tedious specimen preparation, and poor accuracy [7, 8] (as shown in Figure 2.3).

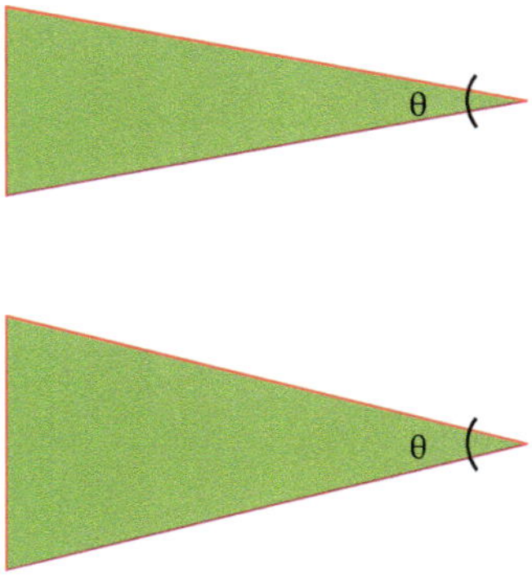


**Figure 2.3** Taper sectioning method – Greater the taper, greater the height variation. *Source:* Bhushan and Talke [7] and Bennett [8].

#### 2.1.2.2 Light-Sectioning Method

The image of a slit (or a straight edge such as a razor blade) is thrown onto the surface at an incident angle of 45°. The reflected image will appear as a straight line if the surface is smooth, and as an undulating line if the surface is rough. The relative vertical magnification of the profile is the cosecant of the angle of incidence, in this case 1.4. Lateral resolution is about 0.5 μm. An automated system for three-dimensional (3D) measurement of surface roughness was described by Uchida et al. (1979) [9]. Their system consists of using the optical system to project the incident slit beam and then observing the image with an industrial television camera projected through a microscope; the table for the test surface is driven by a stepping motor [10] (as shown in Figure 2.4).

#### 2.1.2.3 Specular Reflection Methods

Gloss or specular reflectance (sometimes referred to as sheen or luster) is a surface property of the material, namely, the refractive index and surface roughness. Fresnel's equations provide a relationship between refractive index and reflectance. Surface roughness scatters the reflected light, thus affecting the specular reflectance. Commercial instruments following the general approach are sometimes called specular glossmeters. The first glossmeter was used in the 1920s. A glossmeter detects the specular reflectance (or gloss) of the test surface (of typical size of 50 × 50 mm), which is simply the fraction of the incident light reflected from a surface. Measured specular reflectance is assigned a gloss number. The gloss number is defined as the degree to which the finish of the surface approaches that of the theoretical gloss standard, which is the perfect mirror, assigned a value of 1000 [10, 11] (as shown in Figure 2.5).

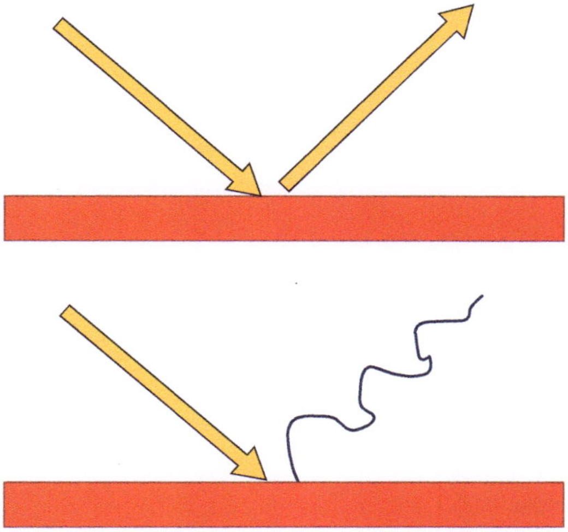

**Figure 2.4** Reflected image appears in a straight line on a smooth surface.

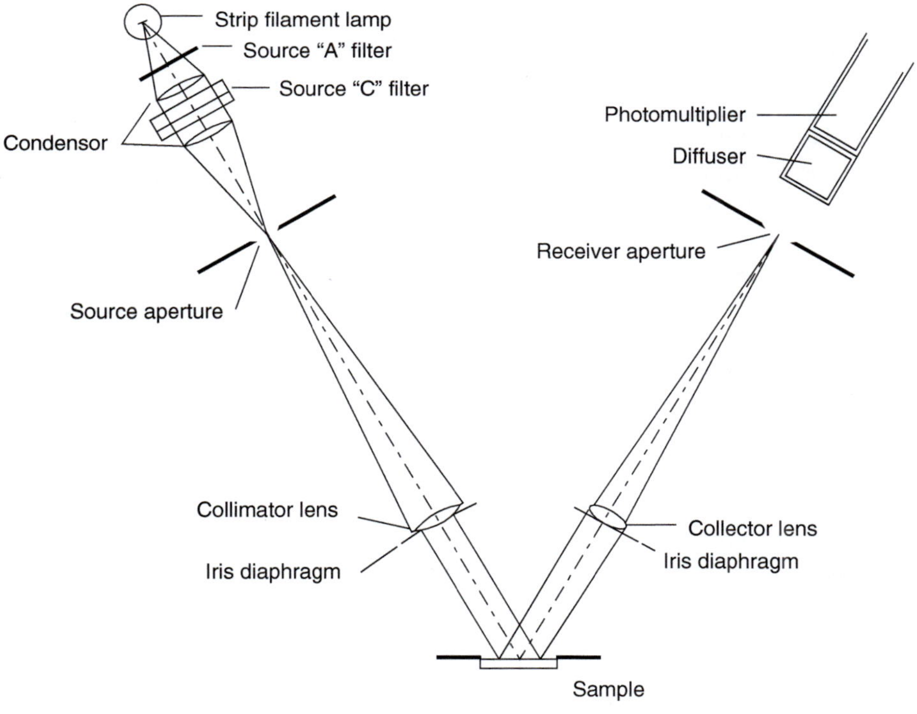


**Figure 2.5** Specular reflection method. *Source:* Bennett and Porteus [10] and Bennett and Mattson [11].

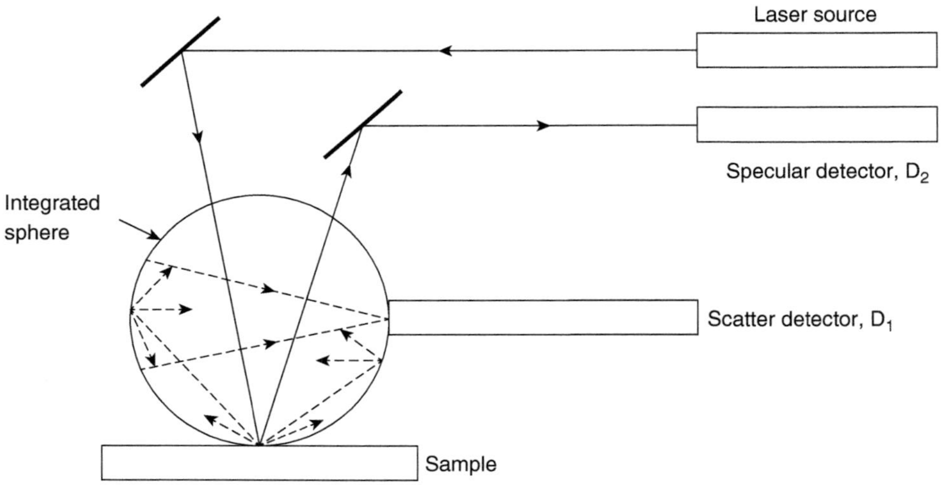


**Figure 2.6** Diffuse reflection method.

#### 2.1.2.4 Diffuse Reflection (Scattering) Methods

Vision depends on diffuse reflection or scattering. Texture, defects, and contamination cause scattering. It is difficult to obtain detailed roughness distribution data from the scattering measurements. Its spatial resolution is based on optical beam size, typically 0.1–1 mm in diameter. Because scatterometers measure light reflectance rather than the actual physical distance between the surface and the sensor, they are relatively insensitive to changes in temperature and mechanical or acoustical vibrations, making them extremely stable and robust. To measure large surface areas, traditional methods scan the roughness of several, relatively small areas (or sometimes just a single scan line) at a variety of locations on the surface. On the other hand, with scatter meters, the inspection spot is quickly and automatically rastered over a large surface. The scattering is sometimes employed to measure surface texture. This technique is particularly suitable for online roughness measurement during manufacture because it is continuous, fast, noncontacting, nondestructive, and relatively insensitive to the environment [11] (as shown in Figure 2.6).

| Good to Know |
|---|
| Specular reflection reflects all light which arrives from a given direction at the same angle, whereas diffuse reflection reflects that light in a broad range of directions. |

#### 2.1.2.5 Speckle Pattern Method

When a rough surface is illuminated with partially coherent light, the reflected beam consists, in part, of random patterns of bright and dark regions known as speckle. Speckle is the local intensity variation between neighboring points. Speckle is the intensity of noise that is usually averaged out. The technique used to relate speckle and surface roughness is the speckle pattern correlation measurement. Here, two speckle patterns are obtained from the test surface by illuminating it with different angles of incidence or different wavelengths of light. Correlation properties of the speckle patterns are then studied by recording the patterns. Goodman (1963) [12] and others have shown that the degree of correlation between speckle patterns depends strongly on the surface roughness ($\sigma$) [8–11].

| Good to Know |
|---|
| Light in which the phases of all electromagnetic waves at each point on a line normal to the direction of the beam are identical. **Coherent light** is usually monochromatic |

#### 2.1.2.6 Optical Interference Methods

Optical interferometry is a valuable technique for measuring surface shape, on both a macroscopic and microscopic scale (Tolansky, 1973) [13]. The traditional technique involves looking at the interference fringes and determining how much they depart from being straight and equally spaced. With suitable computer analysis, these can be used to completely characterize a surface. Bennett (1976) [14] developed an interferometric system employing multiple-beam fringes of equal chromatic order (FECO). FECO are formed when a collimated beam of white light undergoes multiple reflections between two partially silvered surfaces, one of which is the surface whose profile is being measured and the other is a super-smooth reference surface. Based upon a television camera for the detection of the positional displacement of the fringes, this technique has yielded accuracies of $\sigma$ on the order of 0.80 nm for the measurement of surface profiles.

Lateral resolution of this system has been reported to be between 2 and 4 µm, over a 1 mm profile length [8–11].

#### 2.1.2.7 A Commercial Digital Optical Profiler

Figure shows a schematic of a commercial phase-shifting/vertical sensing interference microscope. For smooth surfaces, the phase-shifting mode is used since it gives subnanometer height resolution capability (as shown in Figure 2.7).

For rough surfaces up to 500-µm surface height variations, the vertical scanning coherence sensing technique is used, which gives an approximately 3-nm height resolution. The instrument operates with one of several interchangeable magnification objectives. Each objective contains an interferometer, consisting of a reference mirror and beams splitter, which produces interference fringes when light reflected off the reference mirror recombines with light reflected off the sample. Determination of surface height using phase-shifting interferometry typically involves the sequential shifting of the phase of one beam of the interferometer relative to the other beam by known amounts, and measuring the resulting interference pattern irradiance. Using a minimum of three frames of intensity data, the phase is calculated and is then used to calculate the surface height variations over a surface.

The surface is profiled vertically so that each point on the surface produces an interference signal and the exact vertical position where each signal reaches its maximum amplitude can be located. To obtain the location of the peak, and hence the surface height information, this irradiance signal is detected using a charge-coupled-device (CCD) array.

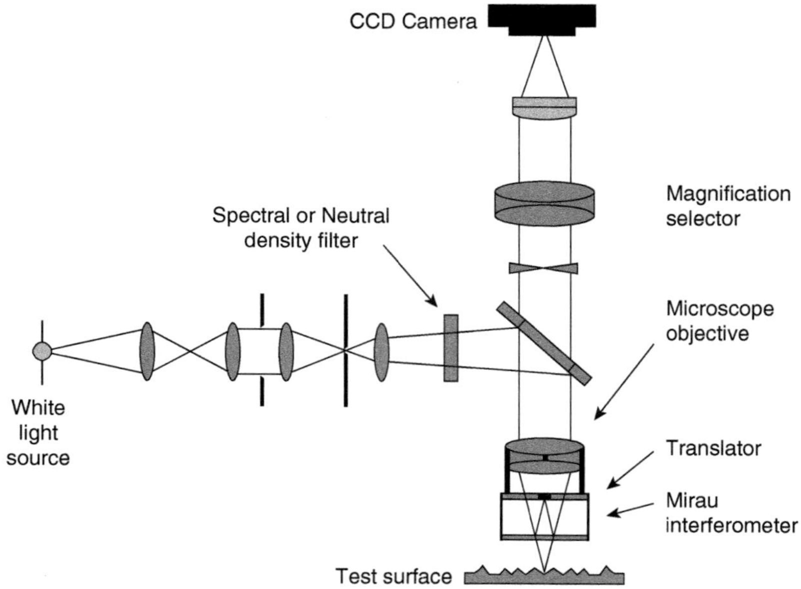


**Figure 2.7** Schematic diagram of a digital profilometer.

The instrument starts the measurement sequence by focusing above the top of the surface being profiled and quickly scanning downward. The signal is sampled at fixed intervals, such as every 50–100 nm, as the sample path is varied. The motion can be accomplished using a piezoelectric transducer. Low-frequency and degree of conversion (DC) signal components are removed from the signal by digital high band-pass filtering. The signal is next rectified by square-law detection and digitally low-pass filtered. The peak of the low-pass filter output is located, and the vertical position corresponding to the peak is noted. Frames of interference data imaged by a video camera are captured and processed by high-speed digital signal processing hardware. As the system scans downward, an interference signal for each point on the surface is formed. A series of advanced algorithms are used to precisely locate the peak of the interference signal for each point on the surface. Each point is processed in parallel, and a 3D map is obtained.

Major advantages of this technique are that its noncontact and 3D measurements can be made rapidly without moving the sample or the measurement tool. One of the limitations of these instruments is that they can only be used for surfaces with similar optical properties [11].

#### 2.1.2.8 Scanning Probe Microscopy (SPM) Methods

The family of instruments based on scanning tunneling microscopy (STM) and atomic force microscopy (AFM) is called SPMs [15, 16].

#### 2.1.2.9 Scanning Tunneling Microscopy (STM)

In 1981, Dr. Gerd Binnig, Heinrich Rohrer and their colleagues introduced vacuum tunneling combined with lateral scanning. Their instrument is called the STM. The vacuum provides the ideal barrier for tunneling. The lateral scanning allows one to image surfaces

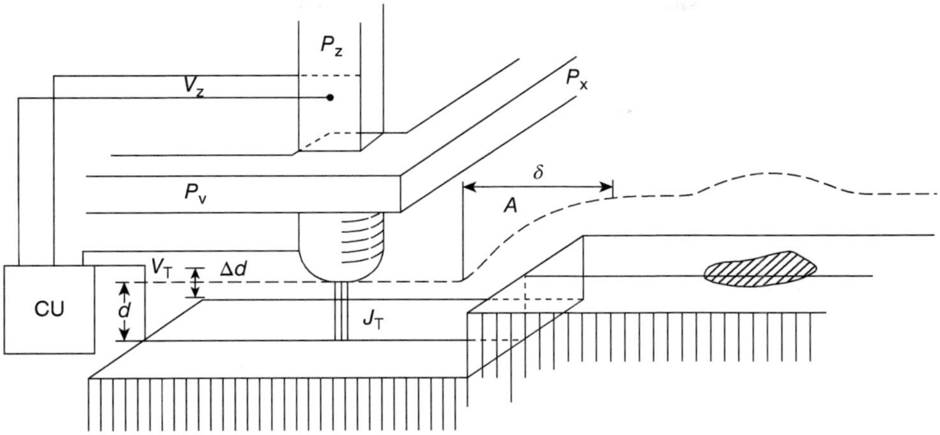


**Figure 2.8** Schematic diagram of scanning tunneling microscope-Px, Py.

with exquisite resolution, laterally <1 nm and vertically <0.1 nm, sufficient to define the position of single atoms. The very high vertical resolution of the STM is obtained because the tunnel current varies exponentially with the distance between the two electrodes, that is, the metal tip and the scanned surface.

STM is the first instrument capable of directly obtaining 3D images of solid surfaces with atomic resolution [16].

The principle of STM is straightforward. A sharp metal tip (one electrode of the tunnel junction) is brought close enough (0.3–1 nm) to the surface to be investigated (second electrode) that, at a convenient operating voltage (10 mV to 2 V), the tunneling current varies from 0.2 to 10 nA, which is measurable. The tip is scanned over a surface at a distance of 0.3–1 nm, while the tunnel current between it and the surface is sensed [16, 17] (as shown in Figure 2.8).

A 1-mm-diameter solid rod, ground at one end at roughly 90°, yields overall tip radii of only a few hundred nanometers, but with closest protrusion of rather sharp microtips on the relatively dull end yields a lateral resolution of about 2 nm. Sharpening of the tips by gently touching the surface brings the resolution down to the 1-nm range; by applying high fields (on the order of 108 V/cm) during, for example, half an hour, resolutions considerably below 1 nm can be reached.

The STM operates in both the "constant height" and "constant current" modes depending on a parameter selection in the control panel. In the constant current mode, the feedback gains are set high, the tunneling tip closely tracks the sample surface, and the variation in the tip height required to maintain constant tunneling current is measured by the change in the voltage applied to the piezo tube. In the constant height mode, the feedback gains are set low, the tip remains at a nearly constant height as it sweeps over the sample surface, and the tunneling current is imaged. A 3D picture [$z(x, y)$] of a surface consists of multiple scans [$z(x)$] displayed laterally from each other in the y direction. Thus, the height data may not be a direct representation of the texture of the surface of the sample [18].

**Good to Know**

The principle of electron tunneling was proposed by Giaever (1960) [19]. He envisioned that if a potential difference is applied to two metals separated by a thin insulating film, the current will flow because of the ability of electrons to penetrate a potential barrier. To be able to measure a tunneling current, the two metals must be spaced no more than 10 nm apart.

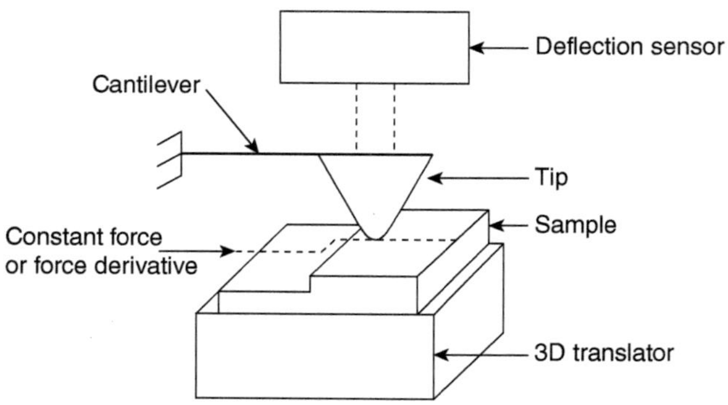


**Figure 2.9** Schematic diagram of atomic force microscope. *Source:* Binnig and Rohrer [18] and Martin et al. [20].

#### 2.1.2.10 Atomic Force Microscopy (AFM)

In 1985, Gerd Binnig and his colleagues developed an instrument called the atomic force microscope, capable of investigating surfaces of both conductors and insulators on an atomic scale. Like the STM, the AFM relies on a scanning technique to produce very high-resolution, 3D images of sample surfaces [18, 20] (as shown in Figure 2.9).

AFM measures ultrasmall forces (<1 nN) present between the AFM tip surface and a sample surface. These small forces are measured by measuring the motion of a very flexible cantilever beam having an ultrasmall mass. In the operation of high-resolution AFM, the sample is generally scanned instead of the tip as an STM. The AFM combines the principles of the STM and the stylus profiler. In the AFM, the force between the sample and tip is detected rather than the tunneling current to sense the proximity of the tip to the sample. A sharp tip at the end of a cantilever is brought into contact with a sample surface by moving the sample with piezoelectric scanners. During initial contact, the atoms at the end of the tip experience a very weak repulsive force due to electronic orbital overlap with the atoms in the sample surface. The force acting on the tip causes a lever deflection which is measured by tunneling, capacitive, or optical detectors such as laser interferometry. The deflection can be measured to within ±0.02 nm, so for a typical lever force constant at 10 N/m, a force as low as 0.2 nN (corresponding normal pressure ~200 MPa for a $Si_3N_4$ tip with a radius of about 50 nm against single-crystal silicon) could be detected [20, 21]

This operational mode is referred to as "repulsive mode" or "contact mode", alternative is to use "attractive force imaging" or "noncontact imaging," in which the tip is brought into close proximity (within a few nanometers) to, and not in contact with, the sample. A very weak van der Waals attractive force is present at the tip–sample interface. Although, in this technique, the normal pressure exerted at the interface is zero (desirable to avoid any surface deformation), it is slow and difficult to use.

In either mode, surface topography is generated by laterally scanning the sample under the tip while simultaneously measuring the separation-dependent force or force gradient (derivative) between the tip and the surface. The force gradient is obtained by vibrating the cantilever [16] and measuring the shift of resonance frequency of the cantilever. To obtain topographic information, the interaction force is either recorded directly or used as a control parameter for a feedback circuit that maintains the force or force derivative at a constant value. Force derivative is normally tracked in noncontact imaging [21].

With AFM operated in the contact mode, topographic images with a vertical resolution of <0.1 nm (as low as 0.01 nm) and a lateral resolution of about 0.2 nm have been obtained. With a 0.01-nm displacement sensitivity, 10 nN to 1 pN forces are measurable. These forces are comparable to the forces associated with chemical bonding, e.g., 0.1 μN for an ionic bond and 10 pN for a hydrogen bond [21].

## 2.2 Water Sorption and Solubility

Restorative dental composites are becomingly more popular and extensively used in dentistry due to their esthetic and good physical and mechanical properties. However, in a wet oral environment, the composites may absorb water or other liquids such as saliva, food components or beverages which can have an appreciable influence on the degradation of dental composite. Excessive liquid uptake may produce deleterious effects on the structure and function of the resin, as these can reduce the mechanical and physical properties that lead to a shortened service life of dental restoration.

Disc-shaped specimens are prepared. The specimens are stored in oven drying at 37 °C for 24 hours, and their masses are measured using analytical balance with a precision 0.001 g. For determining the volume of specimen, the diameter and thickness of each specimen are measured by a digital caliper with a precision 0.001 mm at three points and the mean value is obtained. The specimens are then individually placed in a sealed plastic container containing about 10 ml of immersion media (distilled water, coke and orange juice) at 37 °C. At fixed time intervals (15, 35, 155, 320, 785, etc. min), the specimens are removed, blotted dry to remove excess liquid, weighed and returned to the liquid bath. The sorption equilibrium assumed to be achieved after constant mass ($m2$) was observed at 30 days. The specimens are then reconditioned in a drying oven and weighed during desorption period of 40 days to obtain a constant mass, $m3$.

$$\text{Water sorption} = \left(m2 - m3\right) / V$$
$$\text{Solubility} = \left(m1 - m3\right) / V$$

where $m1$ is the conditioned mass, $m2$ is the mass of specimen after 40 days immersion, and $m3$ is the mass of the reconditioned specimen [22].

## 2.3 Viscosity

Viscosity is the resistance of fluids (liquid or gas) to flow. The physical factors that govern the penetration of restorative materials into the capillary pores of the etched enamel have to be investigated; hence, viscosity is an important parameter.

The formula for viscosity is Shear stress/shear strain. The unit of viscosity is poise.

A viscometer (also called viscosimeter) is an instrument used to measure the viscosity of a fluid. For liquids with viscosities which vary with flow conditions, an instrument called a rheometer is used. Thus, a rheometer can be considered as a special type of viscometer. Viscometers only measure under one flow condition. The drag caused by relative motion of the fluid and a surface is a measure of the viscosity [23].

### 2.3.1 U-Tube Viscometers

These devices are also known as glass capillary viscometers or Ostwald viscometers, named after Wilhelm Ostwald. In one arm of the U is a vertical section of precise narrow bore (the capillary). There are two bulbs, one is positioned higher than the other. The liquid is drawn into the upper bulb by suction and then allowed to flow down through the capillary into the lower bulb. Two marks (one above and one below the upper bulb) indicate a known volume. The time taken for the level of the liquid to pass between these marks is proportional to the kinematic viscosity.

The time required for the test liquid to flow through a capillary of a known diameter of a certain factor between two marked points is measured. By multiplying the time taken by the factor of the viscometer, the kinematic viscosity is obtained [24] (as shown in Figure 2.10).

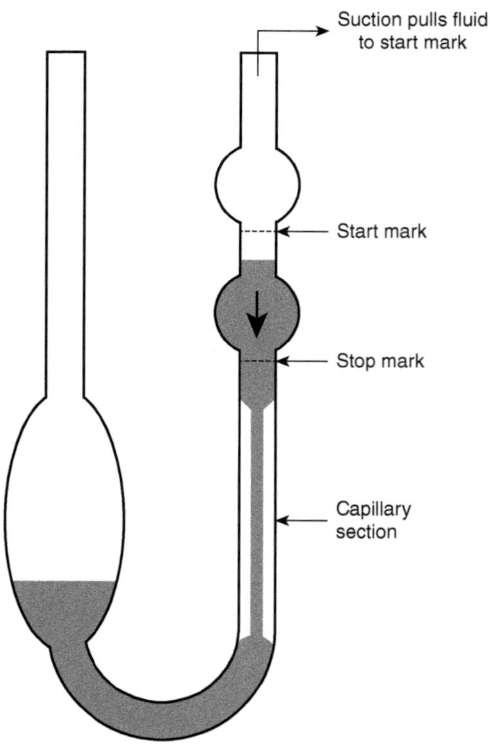


**Figure 2.10** Schematic diagram of a U tube viscometer. *Source:* Based on Dauvillier et al. [24].

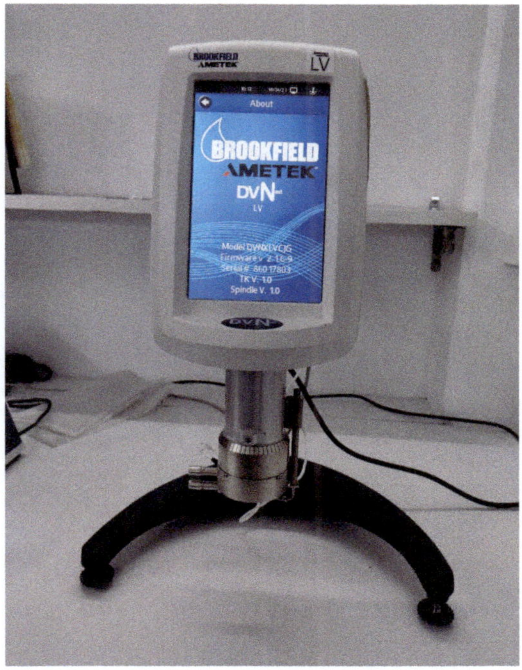


**Figure 2.11** Schematic diagram of a falling sphere viscometer.

### 2.3.2 Falling Sphere Viscometers

In this type, the fluid is stationary in a vertical glass tube. A sphere of known size and density is allowed to descend through the liquid. If correctly selected, it reaches terminal velocity, which can be measured by the time it takes to pass two marks on the tube. Knowing the terminal velocity, the size and density of the sphere, and the density of the liquid, Stokes' law can be used to calculate the viscosity of the fluid. A series of steel ball bearings of different diameters are normally used in the classic experiment to improve the accuracy of the calculation [25].

### 2.3.3 Brookfield's Viscometer

This is based on the principle of rotational viscometry. A calibrated spring is used to apply the torque to a spindle immersed in test fluid. The deflection of the spring measures the viscous drag of the fluid against the spindle. As the liquid to be tested is introduced between the cone and the plate, a resistance to the cone rotation is produced. This is the shear stress of the fluid (as shown in Figure 2.11).

## 2.4 Surface Tension

The measurement of contact angles at the solid–air–liquid meeting point is a widely known technique used to investigate the wettability of solid surfaces [26]. The values obtained depend on the kind of surface topography, surface tension of the liquid and surface energy

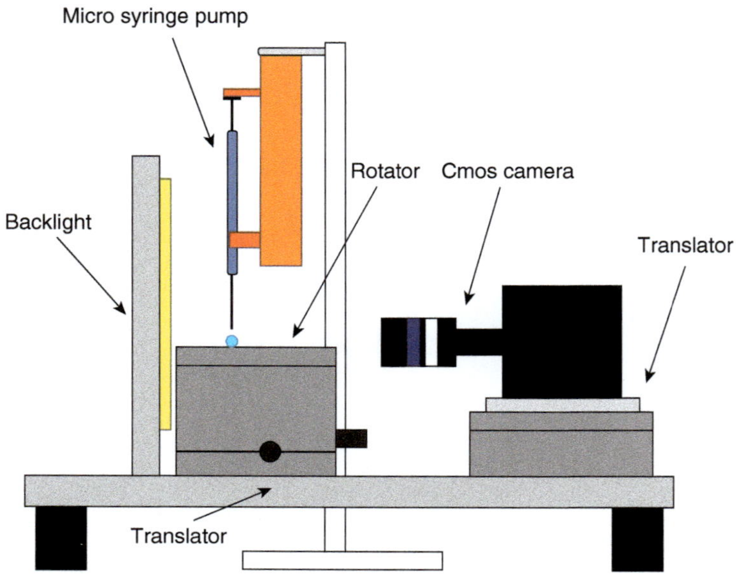


**Figure 2.12** Goniometer.

of the solid substrate [26, 27]. Thus, the relative wetting characteristics of a liquid–solid interface can be inferred by contact angle measurements (as shown in Figure 2.12).

Scientists commonly use an optical goniometer/tensiometer to measure the surface tension and interfacial tension of a liquid using the pendant or sessile drop methods. A drop is produced and captured using a CCD camera. The drop profile is subsequently extracted, and softwares are used which use the theoretical Young–Laplace equation to the experimental drop profile. The surface tension can then be calculated from the fitted parameters [28].

The contact angle method is relatively simple, very useful and highly sensitive to investigate the interfacial phenomena. The contact angle is the angle between the surface of the wetted solid and a line tangent to the curved surface of the drop at the point of three-phase contact. Water (distilled many times) and methylene iodide (Kemphasol, Bombay) are used for the analyses of samples. Measurements are carried out on samples of dimension $6 \times 2 \times 0.3\,\text{mm}^3$ at room temperature in closed chambers. The volume of the sessile drop is maintained as 5 µl in all cases using a microsyringe. For accuracy, measurements are repeated 5–10 times on different pieces of the same sample [28, 29].

When a liquid drop is brought onto the surface of a solid, the contact of liquid/solid reaches an equilibrium condition and we say the liquid drop is in a static state. Whether it will wet the surface or not depends on the relative magnitudes of the molecular forces that exist within the liquid (cohesive) and between the liquid and the solid (adhesive). The angle with which the liquid subtends the solid is known as the contact angle (θ). Such a contact angle is used to characterize the wettability of a liquid on a solid surface. Because the contact angle ranges from 0 to 180°, there are two extreme cases. If the contact angle is equal to 0°, i.e., a liquid film is formed on a solid surface, then we can say that a perfect wetting occurs. The other case is that the contact angle is equal to 180°, i.e., a perfect liquid sphere is set on the solid surface [29] (as shown in Figure 2.13).

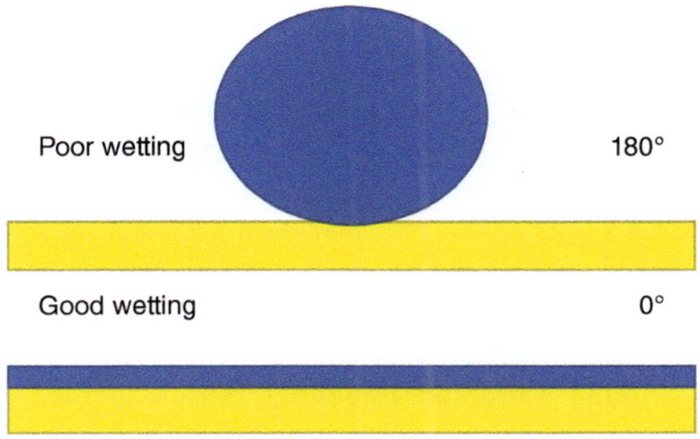


**Figure 2.13** Diagrammatic representation of contact angle of a liquid on a surface.

## 2.5 Degree of Conversion

DC is clinically significant as it affects the strength, hardness, elastic modulus, dimensional stability, solubility, water sorption, and color stability as well as biocompatibility of restorative materials [30]. Higher DC implies larger polymeric molecules that yield better physical properties and less free monomer that may leach from the restoration and potentially exert cytotoxic and genotoxic effects [30]. Conventional composite materials usually reach a DC of about 50–75%. For bulk-fill materials, DC values ranging from 50% to 79% have been reported. Some authors suggest a DC of 55% as a minimal value for clinical success [30, 31]. Although the exact threshold DC value required for clinical success of a restoration cannot be determined, DC is a useful predictor of a restoration's physical and mechanical properties, as well as biocompatibility. To assess the DC, direct and indirect methods can be used. Direct methods based on vibrational spectroscopy are considered more accurate because they directly quantify the amount of unreacted C=C bonds [32]. Indirect methods of DC determination correlate the DC and microhardness values and may prove inaccurate. Although Fourier transform infrared (FTIR) spectroscopy has been traditionally used for DC assessment, Raman spectroscopy provides an alternative method that may, in some experimental designs, prove simpler and more adaptive than FTIR [33]. Sample preparation for Raman spectroscopy has no specific requirements, and the sample can be used as-made, i.e., no additional sample processing is required. In addition to easier sample handling, Raman also enables multiple measurements on the same sample due to the non-destructive sample preparation. While FTIR spectroscopy measures the absorption of incident radiation, Raman is based on the inelastic scattering phenomenon. Molecules in the sample are excited to a virtual energy state by laser light and then relaxed to a molecular vibrational state followed by emission of photons with energy different from energy of the incident photon. A Raman photon is emitted if a molecule undergoes a transition to a higher vibrational energy state than its original state (Stokes-Raman), or to a lower energy vibrational state (Anti-Stokes Raman) [32, 33]. The energy spectrum of emitted photons is determined by vibrational energy states that are characteristic for specific functional groups and chemical bonds. As in FTIR spectroscopy, the band at 1640 c/m is assigned to the vibrations of C=C bonds and its relative change in intensity before and after curing is used to calculate the DC. When used for the DC assessment of dental composites, Raman and FTIR spectroscopy yield similar results [34].

## 2.6 Microleakage

Microleakage is defined as the movement of bacteria, fluids, molecules, or ions between the tooth and restorations of any type. In restorative dentistry, microleakage can occur between the tooth and restoration, tooth and bonding agent, restoration and bonding agent interface and also between the tooth surface and the prosthetic crown. In endodontics, microleakage between the obturating material and the root dentin can ultimately disrupt the fluid tight seal and can lead to root canal failure. Several techniques have been developed to study marginal permeability at the interface between the tooth and the restoration. The margins of restorations are not fixed neither are they inert with impenetrable borders, as the clinician would like to view them. They "possess dynamic micro crevices which contain a busy traffic of ions and molecules" according to Myers in 1966.

Microleakage often results in dentinal hypersensitivity by creating a direct communication between oral fluids and the pulp, secondary caries, pulpal pathology and marginal discoloration around restorations. Microleakage in endodontics can ultimately result in reinfection or failure of the root canal treatment [35, 36].

### 2.6.1 Methods Used for Detection of Microleakage

Many techniques have been devised to test the cavity-sealing properties of restorations.

**The various methods include** [35, 36]

- Use of dyes
- Chemical tracers
- Radioactive isotopes
- Bacteria
- Air pressure
- Neutron activation analysis
- Artificial caries
- Scanning electron microscopy (SEM)
- Electrical conductivity
- Fluid filtration

Leakage tests can be subdivided into old and contemporary methods. Old methods were used to test the presence of gaps and the sealing ability of different restorative materials. These methods included air pressure, fluid filtration, neutron activation, electrical conductivity, bacteria, and artificial caries. Contemporary methods include radioactive methods, chemical tracers, dye methods, SEM, confocal laser scanning microscopy and 3D methods such as micro-CT and Optical Coherence Tomography (OCT).

### 2.6.2 Air Pressure

Air pressure was introduced for detection of marginal leakage by Harper in 1912 [37]. He constructed class 2 amalgam restorations in a steel dye, delivered air under pressure to the floor of the cavity, and examined the restoration under water. Microscopic examination of the release of air bubbles from the margin of the submerged restoration provided a subjective view of the marginal seal. This method proved to be a valuable technique for comparing the sealing properties of different amalgams as well as cements [37].

**Advantages**:

- Results can be quantified.
- Specimen destruction is not required in this method.

**Disadvantages**:

- detects leakage pathways from the floor to the margin of the cavity
- does not take into account the drying effect of compressed air which is passing through the restoration.

### 2.6.3 Fluid Filtration

The fluid filtration method was developed by Derkson et al. and modified by Wu et al. for use in endodontics. In the fluid filtration technique, the coronal or apical tip of the sample is attached to a micropipette which has been filled with liquid. Using a syringe, the water is sucked back approximately 3 mm into the open end of the glass capillary, creating an air bubble in the capillary tube. The whole setup is then placed in a water bath at a constant temperature and pressure. The amount of bubble displacement during a specified period of time is measured, which is a sign of the amount of liquid passage through the sample and present the microleakage of that sample and is calculated in μl/min [38].

**Advantages**:

- The samples are not destroyed
- The results obtained are precise and quantitative.

**Disadvantages**:

- Any change in temperature and pressure can affect the result.

### 2.6.4 Neutron Activation Analysis

Neutron activation analysis involves immersing restored teeth in an aqueous solution of a nonradioactive manganese salt. All of the salt adhering to the outside of the tooth is then removed, and the whole tooth is placed in the core of a nuclear reactor. This results in the nonradioactive $Mn^{55}$ being activated to $Mn^{56}$, and the X-ray emission of $Mn^{56}$ formed during irradiation is then measured. The number of radioactive counts is proportional to the uptake of Mn per tooth [39].

**Advantages**:

- Results can be quantified.

**Disadvantages**:

- Inability to identify the points where the restoration has leaked.
- The experimental setup involves high cost

- The procedure is complex and involves a combined effort from nuclear scientists and dental researchers
- The process involves radiation hazard

### 2.6.5 Electrical Conductivity

A conductimetric technique to evaluate changes in the dimensions of the cavity wall/restoration interspace using an electrochemical cell was developed by Jacobson and von Fraunhofer in 1975. This technique involves the use of glass tubes of 4 mm internal diameter and cut into lengths of 15 mm because glass ($9.7 \times 10^{-6}$/°C) has a similar coefficient of thermal expansion to that of tooth substance ($11.4 \times 10^{-6}$/°C). The floor of the "cavity" is formed by a nickel-plated brass electrode. After inserting the material, 4 mm of the glass tube is immersed in a 1% solution of lactic acid. A lead from the brass electrode is connected to one terminal of a 5 V power source, while the other terminal of the circuit is connected through a series of resistances to a reference electrode that is formed by a nickel-plated brass rod. The circuit is completed when the interspace between the test material and glass is occupied by electrolytes. Any change in the current passing through this electrochemical cell reflects changes in the dimensions of the interspace. Since the dimensions of the cavities are constant, the dimensional changes of the materials themselves are observed through measurements of the potential change in the experimental circuit. The test method does not demand destruction of the specimen and thus allows changes in the dimensions of the interspace to be followed through different time periods. It does not take into account the dielectric properties of the restorative material or that these (especially in the case of glass-ionomer polyalkenoate cements) may change with time as setting reactions continue. This method, therefore, seems to lack clinical realism [40].

**Limitations**

- A major limitation of the technique is that it cannot be used to study microleakage properties of metallic restorations.

### 2.6.6 Bacteria

Bacteria have also been used in the study of microleakage. Probably the earliest such study was in 1929 when Fraser tested cements and restorative materials to determine whether they would allow bacteria to pass through or around them. Later, workers investigating the marginal seal of acrylic restorations placed filled teeth in broth cultures. The filling materials were subsequently removed and dentin shavings from the base of the cavity cultured. This provided purely qualitative results, depending mainly upon the presence or absence of bacteria in part of the dentin shavings examined. Mortensen et al. (1965) [41] developed a method for isolating the filled crown of a tooth from its root using a plastic tube sealed with epoxy resin. Broth inoculated with a bacterial culture was placed over the crown, while sterile broth was placed in contact with the root of the tooth. Microleakage was diagnosed if the sterile broth turned cloudy [37, 38].

**Advantages**:

- The technique is more clinically relevant

**Disadvantages**:

- The results can be assessed qualitatively
- The method is unable to detect small gaps. It can detect gaps measuring 0.5–1 μm or larger

### 2.6.7 Artificial Caries

Artificial secondary caries-like lesions have been produced in vitro using either bacterial cultures or a chemical system-the acidified gel technique. In 1967, Ellis and Brown, using a bacterial technique to produce artificial secondary caries at the interface of the amalgam restoration and the tooth, linked the development of carious lesions to microleakage. The histological appearance of lesions under polarized light shows two parts: an "outer lesion" and a "cavity wall" lesion. The outer lesion represents the features of primary attack, while the inner cavity wall lesion represents the microleakage of ions from the caries inducing medium into the tooth restoration interface [42, 43]

**Advantages**:

- Microleakage may be linked directly to secondary caries.
- quantification of results can be obtained using this method.
- Degree of demineralization can also be assessed quantitatively

**Disadvantages**:

- It is not appropriate for examining marginal leakage where the cavity preparation includes acid etching.

### 2.6.8 Radioactive Tracers

Another common method for detecting leakage patterns involves the use of radioactive isotopes. The use of isotopes permits detection of minute amounts of leakage, as the smaller isotope molecules measure only 40 nm compared to the smaller dye particles (120 nm). The tracers that have been used are $Ca^{45}$, $C^{14}$, $I^{131}$ $P^{31}$, $S^{35}$ and $Na^{22}$ [44]. This method for detecting microleakage in vitro involves the use of extracted restored teeth. The roots and crowns of the teeth are painted with varnish except for the surface immediately adjacent to the experimental restoration. This is to prevent leakage through the root canal, cracks in the enamel, or exposed dentin, which can obliterate the true picture of marginal adaptation. The sealed teeth are immersed in the isotope solution for several hours. After removal from the isotope, the teeth are subjected to prolonged rinsing before ground longitudinal sections are made through the restoration. The samples are placed on a photographic film to generate an autoradiograph that indicates the presence and location of any radioactive isotope that has penetrated between the restoration and the cavity wall. However, the results are evaluated by subjective scoring [44–46].

**Advantages**:

- The method can detect leakage in minute amounts.
- The use of isotopes allows greater penetration into crevices than dyes.

**Disadvantages**:

- The results are subjective in nature thereby dependent on observer interpretation.
- A high-energy isotope produces more scatter on the film leading to an increase in apparent leakage.
- The method is expensive and technique sensitive.
- All precautionary measures are to be taken to satisfy safety requirements.

### 2.6.9 Chemical Tracers

Kornfield (1953) [47] described a technique for assessing leakage around acrylic restorations by incorporating lead glass in the acrylic, so that when immersed in a solution of barium sulfide, areas of marginal discoloration indicated leakage. The silver nitrate method of measuring microleakage is an acceptable technique. It is, however, a severe test because the silver ion is extremely small (0.059 nm) when compared to the size of a typical bacterium (0.5–1.0 μm) and thus is more penetrative. Therefore, it may be assumed that any system that prevents the leakage of the silver ion will also prevent leakage of bacteria. A 50% silver nitrate solution is commonly used to immerse the in vitro model, which later is reacted with a photographic developing solution such as benzene 1, 4-diol (hydroquinone). Other investigators used 1% silver chloride because the electrochemical technique provided no visual indication of what was occurring. This silver-staining technique gave a discrete, high-contrast marking of the restoration/dentin interface [48, 49].

**Advantages**:

- Depth of penetration is much better defined
- It is a more objective method

**Disadvantages**:

- Results can be evaluated subjectively
- The process demands destruction of the specimen

### 2.6.10 Dyes

The use of organic dyes as tracers is one of the oldest and most common methods of detecting leakage in vitro. As far back as 1874, King used blue ink and Tomes (1875) [50] used draper's ink in leakage studies. In 1895, Fletcher used dyes to study the shrinkage of dental amalgam [51].

**The following are the list of dyes commonly used**:

- Eosin
- Methylene blue
- Methyl violet

- Hematoxylin
- Mercuric chloride
- Prontosil soluble red
- Aniline dye
- Basic fuchsin
- Chromotrope 2R
- Crystal violet dye
- Fluorescent dye (fluorescein)

In general, this method for detecting microleakage in vitro involves placing a restoration in an extracted tooth and immersing it in a dye solution, after coating the unfilled parts of the tooth with a waterproof varnish. After a predetermined time period, the specimen is removed, washed, and sectioned before visual examination to establish the extent of penetration of dye around the filling. Christen and Mitchell in 1966 found that different concentrations of dyes can vary in penetration time between five minutes to over one hour. Fluorescent dyes are found to be particularly useful as tracers because they are detectable in dilute concentration, inexpensive, and being nontoxic can be used safely for clinical as well as laboratory investigations [52, 53]. Some dyes such as basic fuchsin have been shown to bind preferentially with carious dentin. Dyes that exhibit a propensity for bonding to tooth structure or restorative material under investigation can potentially demonstrate a wider and deeper gap than actually exists. The assessment of the restoration as a whole is difficult because most sectioning is done on class 5 restorations in the sagittal plane. Dye-penetration studies demand destruction of the specimen and thus make it impossible to use fully quantitative techniques for evaluation [53]. However, others have suggested that dye penetration is nondestructive, thus allowing longitudinal study of restoration margins [54]. Dentin permeability is also another factor to be considered. The diameter of the dentinal tubules and the number of tubules per unit surface increase as the tubules converge toward the pulp. Practically, it is undesirable to use any dye particle that has a diameter greater than that of the internal diameter of the dentinal tubules (1–4 μm). Therefore, leakage studies in dentin will show some degree of dentin staining that should be differentiated from actual microleakage between the cavity and restoration. It has been suggested that dentin involvement might be used as a relative indicator of marginal leakage [54, 55].

**Advantages**:

- Microleakage is detectable in dilute concentration
- It is an inexpensive method

**Disadvantages**:

- Results can be evaluated subjectively
- The method demands destruction of the specimen

| **Good to Know** |
|---|
| The concentrations of dye used ranges between 0.5% and 10%, while the time of immersion of specimens in the dye varies between 4 and 72 hours or more |

### 2.6.11 Dye Extraction Technique

In this method, the teeth are dissolved in acids, releasing all the dyes from the interfacial areas and a spectrophotometer determines the optical density (OD) of the solution. Specimens are coated with nail varnish except for the area of interest. They are placed in 2% methylene blue dye for 72 hours. Then, the specimens are washed with distilled water, the nail varnish removed, and then they were placed in 35% nitric acid for 72 hours. Standard solutions of 1%, 0.5%, 0.005%, 0.002%, 0.001%, and 0.0005% of methylene blue in 35% nitric acid were prepared and stored for 72 hours. The vials are centrifuged at 14 000 rpm for five minutes. The dye absorption is measured by an automatic spectrophotometer at 550 nm using concentrated nitric acid as the blank. The results of the spectrophotometer indicate the light absorption of the methylene blue in the resin-dentin interface which is actually showing the microleakage of the restoration [56].

**Advantage**:

- A quantitative result is obtained.
- Accuracy is high

**Disadvantage**:

- Specimen destruction

None of the methods used for the detection of microleakage is ideal. Probably, the most practical method that provides an acceptable degree of reliability is penetration by tracers. As pointed out previously, tracers have a number of disadvantages. When compared with other methods, however, they provide an effective in vitro method that allows fair comparison between different restorative techniques and materials. Radioactive isotopes have the advantage over dyes as tracers, for their presence can be readily detected in very small concentrations. Bacterial microleakage is best examined in vivo, but conducting strictly controlled in vivo experiments requires large numbers of specimens, is time-consuming, and expensive.

### 2.6.12 Scanning Electron Microscopy (SEM)

The use of SEM provides a means of direct visual observation of the adaptation of restorative materials to cavity margins because of its high magnification and depth of focus. It has been pointed out that the SEM technique can be criticized for its potential for introducing errors and artifacts related to drying, cracking, distortion and sectioning. The technique is limited to the evaluation of teeth outside the oral environment and is not oriented to diffusion and penetration as are most other studies. However, many workers have used SEM to measure gap formation that occurred between the restorations and walls and floor of the preparation. The method of SEM can be improved by the use of replicas. This allows change in the size of marginal defects to be followed on a longitudinal basis and can be applied clinically. Replicas may be repeated many times at different intervals, and this does not change the structures being evaluated. The use of a replica technique may avoid specimen shrinkage, and some of the other artifacts were usually associated with preparation of biological tissue for SEM examination. It is also difficult to quantify SEM results, and the technique is limited to demonstrating marginal defects [57].

**Advantage**:

- Provides means of direct visual observation of the adaptation of restorative materials to cavity margins due to its high magnification (200×–100×) and depth of focus.

**Disadvantage**:

- Drying of specimens, dehydration and embedding of the specimens which is usually needed for SEM analysis may result in artifacts, affecting the image outcomes.
- The sample preparation may also affect the surface morphology resulting interference during observation.

### 2.6.13 Confocal Laser Scanning Microscopy

This technique merges the capabilities of scanning, transmitted and X-ray microscopes and achieves unprecedented resolutions in optically dense materials by implementing the technology of confocal imaging into an electron microscope [58, 59].

**Advantage**:

- High-resolution images are obtained.
- It has the ability to produce images that are acquired point-by-point and then reconstructed in a computer, thereby allowing three-dimensional image reconstruction.
- The use of fluorescent dyes provides better contrast.

**Disadvantage**:

- Thin slices of samples of thickness 0.5 microns need to be prepared with extreme caution in order to avoid chipping of removal of the area of interest.

### 2.6.14 Micro-CT

With the development of micro-computed tomography (μCT), researchers have been capable of evaluating the microleakage of dental restorative materials, and leakage area and volume determined by 3D image analysis have been correlated with a variety of materials. Moreover, μCT has proven to be a powerful and viable technique in determining polymerization shrinkage and microleakage. For the analysis, each teeth needs to be stabilized in the sample holder of the system, the X-ray source is set to 100 kV/100 mA, and a 1 mm aluminum filter is used to scan all samples. Each sample is rotated 360°, with a rotation step of 0.50°. The magnification is set at 20, which results in a pixel size of 9 μm. A software is used in further cone-beam reconstruction of all the projected X-ray images. Each microscan is cropped to have a smaller sample including the regions of interest (ROI). Subsequently, 410–440 micro-CT slices to the 950 slices are selected and saved as Bit-Mapped Pixels (BMP) image files with a resolution of 2000 × 2000 pixels, showing 2D images. Then, these BMP files are exported to CT-Analyser (CTAn) software. A circle ROI is selected on each data set slice by slice. Finally, microleakage volume and percentage (microleakage/ROI × 100) are analyzed [60–63].

**Advantage**:

- 3D analysis of microleakage is possible with this method.

**Disadvantage**:

- High cost of equipment
- Lower precision in comparison to conventional dye penetration observed under a stereomicroscope [64].

### 2.6.15 Optical Coherence Tomography

In dental science, OCT detects qualitative and quantitative morphological changes of dental hard and soft tissues in vivo. Furthermore, OCT can also be used for early diagnosis of dental diseases, including caries, periodontal disease, and oral cancer, because of the excellent spatial resolution. OCT can provide effective information because it is noninvasive and nondestructive and does not expose patients to radiation; in addition, it provides a real-time monitoring method. OCT has high axial resolution of about 10 μm; this allows sufficient information for dental clinical applications such as the diagnosis of crack and microleakage detection.

Using radiographs and clinical examination, the ROIs are chosen and marked for OCT imaging. The scanning probe acquired images on the marked tooth. A metal marker is placed on the probe to ensure complete image acquisition at each rotating scan. The metal has high reflection on the OCT image. The detected light is stable for good image quality with a range of angle. It can differentiate between a sound tooth and a restored tooth [65–67].

**Advantages**:

- It is a noninvasive, nondestructive procedure.
- Allows real-time imaging.
- It allows in vivo identification of microleakage.

**Disadvantages**:

- The equipment is expensive.

| Good to Know |
|---|
| Although there are several techniques for detection of microleakage, the dye techniques are most commonly employed. The highest precision is seen with confocal laser scanning microscopy which can measure up to 100 microns |

## 2.7 Interfacial Adaptation and Film Thickness

One reason for resin-bonded composite, direct restoration failure is postoperative pain or sensitivity. Poor internal adaptation of a resin composite restoration will create gaps between the material and the tooth structure and allow fluid collection. This fluid will move into the dentinal tubules due to pressure changes created during mastication or temperature fluctuations, causing the patient to feel pain. Many factors, including material properties, cavity preparation design, and operative technique, influence the quality of adaptation of resin bonded composite (RBC) restorations. However, polymerization shrinkage and its associated stress are two of the most adverse properties of current materials. Many clinical techniques, such as controlling the curing light intensity, indirect placement of resin restorations, application of a flowable resin liner, and incremental layering techniques, have been introduced to minimize the shrinkage stress and thereby reduce gap formation. However, no method has been shown to be totally effective in abating the effects of polymerization shrinkage. Interfacial adaptation can be assessed by scanning electron microscope, OCT, μCT, and image analysis technique [68, 69].

Film thickness as per ANSI/ADA specification number 96 (ISO 9917-1) is the thickness in micrometers of set cement after 10 minutes of load application. Load is 150 N. It is applied by a flat plate against another flat surface. The thickness should be <25 μm for luting cements [70].

## 2.8 Radiopacity

Briefly, there have been different methods for assessing the radiopacity of dental materials including densitometer, digital, or digitalized radiography by means of an aluminum step wedge or the attenuation coefficient method. According to ISO 4049:2009, a monochromatic X-ray source performing within the range of $65 \pm 5$ kVp using a D-speed and #4 sized film should be applied. Moreover, the step wedge should have a purity of at least 98% aluminum, not consisting of more than 0.1% copper or 1% iron. One-millimeter-thick samples of restorative material should be prepared. In addition, a 12-step wedge (1 mm incremental steps) has to be made from a 93%-pure alumina alloy ingot.

An occlusal phosphor storage plates (PSP) digital sensor can also be used. The captured images are processed by a Digora Panoramic, Cephalometric and Tomographic (PCT) device (Soredex, Tuusula, Finland) with 40–85 μm pixel size, 4–6 lp/mm and 16 bit color depth. Digital radiopacities are measured and read in Digora for Windows 2.5 software (Soredex, Tuusula, Finland) at the program default status with no enhancement or further manipulation of contrast. The radiopacities are measured from five different areas (i.e., four corner poles plus the central area), each with a $40 \times 40$ pixel area, in order to reduce the measurement bias. Then, the average calculated radiopacity of each sample is calculated. Thereafter, the obtained radiopacities are transformed to the final digital radiopacity (absorbance) using the following equation: $A = -\log(T) = -\log(1-G/255)$, where $A$ was the absorbance, $T$ was the transmission, and $G$ was the gray scale (0–255). For each set of exposure time/tube-target distance, the radiopacity of aluminum alloy is plotted against the corresponding thickness and a specific linear model was calculated. Briefly, the $Y = a + bX$ equation is obtained from plotting the radiopacity of aluminum steps against their thickness, where "$Y$" is the radiopacity, "$a$" is the constant of regression, "$b$" is the coefficient of the line and "$X$" is the thickness [71, 72].

**Key Points**

1) Surface roughness, water sorption and solubility, viscosity and surface tension, degree of conversion, microleakage, interfacial adaption and radiopacity are commonly studied physical properties of dental material.
2) Each of these properties requires different experimental setup.
3) Surface roughness of restorative materials has been recognized as a parameter of high clinical relevance for plaque accumulation, staining susceptibility and wear.
4) ISO 4049 is a standard method which is commonly used by researchers to determine water sorption and solubility of restorative dental composites. The standard limits for the water sorption and solubility are 40 and 7.5 $g/mm^3$, respectively.
5) The physical factors that govern the penetration of restorative resins are viscosity, surface tension and contact angle.
6) Degree of conversion is a useful predictor of a restoration's physical and mechanical properties, as well as biocompatibility. To assess the DC, direct and indirect methods can be used. Direct methods based on vibrational spectroscopy are considered more accurate because they directly quantify the amount of unreacted C=C bonds.
7) Microleakage is defined as the movement of bacteria, fluids, molecules or ions between the tooth and restorations of any type. In restorative dentistry, microleakage can occur between the tooth and restoration, tooth and bonding agent, restoration and bonding agent interface and also between the tooth surface and the prosthetic crown. In endodontics, microleakage between the obturating material and the root dentin can ultimately disrupt the fluid tight seal and can lead to root canal failure.

## References


1 Abbott, E.J. and Firestone, F.A. (1933). Specifying surface quality. *Mech. Eng.* 55: 569–572.

2 Rawls, R. (2013). *Phillips' Science of Dental Materials*. St. Louis, MO: Elsevier/Saunders.

3 Sadeghi, M., Deljoo, Z., and Bagheri, R. (2016). The influence of surface polish and beverages on the roughness of nanohybrid and microhybrid resin composite. *J. Dent. Biomater.* 3 (1): 177–185.

4 Thomas, T.R. (1999). *Rough Surfaces*, 2nde. London: Imperial College Press.

5 Anonymous (1975). Instruments for the measurement of surface roughness by profile methods. ISO3274, International Standardization Organization.

6 Anonymous (1985). *Surface Texture (Surface Roughness, Waviness and Lay), NSI/ASME B46.1*. New York, NY: ASME.

7 Bhushan, B. and Talke, F. (1991). Tribology and mechanics of magnetic storage devices. *J. Tribol.* 113 (1): 225–225.

8 Bennett, J. (2004). Surface Roughness and Scattering. *Proc. Manuf. Mach. Tool Conf.* 2004.5: 15–16.

9 Uchida, S., Sato, H., and O-Hori, M. (1979), Two-dimensional measurement of surface roughness by the light sectioning method, *Annals CIRP*, 28, 419–423.

10 Bennett, H.E. and Porteus, J.O. (1961). Relation between surface roughness and specular reflectance at normal incidence. *J. Opt. Soc. Amer.* 51: 123–129.

**11** Bennett, J.M. and Mattson, L. (1989). *Introduction to Surface Roughness and Scattering*. Washington, DC: Optical Society of America.

**12** Goodman, J.W. (1963), *Statistical Properties of Laser Speckle Patterns*, Tech. Rep. No. 2303–1, Stanford Electronics Lab., Palo Alto, CA.

**13** Tolansky, S. (1973), *Introduction to Interferometers*, Wiley, New York.

**14** Bennett, J.M. (1976), Measurement of the rms roughness, autocovariance function and other statistical properties of optical surfaces using a FECO scanning interferometer, *Appl. Opt.*, 15, 2705–2721.

**15** Boyde, A. (1971). Practical problems and methods in the three-dimensional analysis of scanning electron microscope images. Scanning Electron Microscopy, Proceedings of the Third Annual SEM Symposium, IITRI, Chicago, IL, 105–112.

**16** Lange, S.R. and Bhushan, B. (1988). Use of two- and three-dimensional, noncontact surface profiler for tribology applications. *Surf. Topogr.* 1: 277–290.

**17** Anonymous (1992a). *Nanoscope III Scanning Tunneling Microscope*. Santa Barbara, CA: Instruction Manual, Digital Instruments.

**18** Binnig, G. and Rohrer, H. (1983). Scanning tunnelling microscopy. *Surf. Sci.* 126: 236–244.

**19** Giaever, I. (1960), Energy gap in superconductors measured by electron tunnelling, *Phys. Rev. Lett.*, 5, 147–148.

**20** Martin, Y., Williams, C.C., and Wickramasinghe, H.K. (1987). Atomic force microscope-force mapping profiling on a sub 100-A scale. *J. Appl. Phys.* 61: 4723–4729.

**21** Anonymous (1992b). *Nanoscope III Atomic Force Microscope*. Santa Barbara, CA: Instruction Manual, Digital Instruments.

**22** Rahim, T.N.A.T., Mohamad, D., Md Akil, H., and Ab Rahman, I. (2012). Water sorption characteristics of restorative dental composites immersed in acidic drinks. *Dent. Mater.* 28 (6): e63–e70.

**23** Barnes, H.A., Hutton, J.F., and Walters, K. (1989). *An Introduction to Rheology*, 5e, 12. Amsterdam: Elsevier.

**24** Dauvillier, B.S., Feilzer, A.J., De Gee, A.J., and Davidson, C.L. (2000). Visco-elastic parameters of dental restorative materials during setting. *J. Dent. Res.* 79 (3): 818–823.

**25** Mason, W.P. and Hill, M. (1947). Measurement of the viscosity and shear elasticity of liquids by means of a torsionally vibrating crystal. *J. Lubr. Technol.* 69: 359–370.

**26** Rame, E. and Garoff, S. (1996). Microscopic and macroscopic dynamic interface shapes and the interpretation of dynamic contact angles. *J. Colloid Interface Sci.* 177 (1): 234–244.

**27** Silikas, N., Kavvadia, K., Eliades, G., and Watts, D. (2005). Surface characterization of modern resin composites: a multitechnique approach. *Am. J. Dent.* 18 (2): 95–100.

**28** Jasper, W.J. and Rasipuram, S. (2017). Relationship between contact angle and contact line radius for micro to atto [10−6 to 10−18] liter size oil droplets. *J. Mol. Liq.* 248: 920–926.

**29** de Gennes, P.G. (1985). Wetting: statics and dynamics. *Rev. Mod. Phys.* 57 (3): 827–863.

**30** Calixto, L.R., Lima, D.M., Queiroz, R.S. et al. (2008, 1365). Curing depth of composite resin light cured by LED and halogen light-curing units. *Laser Phys.* 18: -1369.

**31** Soares, L.E., Liporoni, P.C., and Martin, A.A. (2007). The effect of soft-start polymerization by second generation LEDs on the degree of conversion of resin composite. *Oper. Dent.* 32: 160–165.

**32** Stahl, F., Ashworth, S.H., Jandt, K.D., and Mills, R.W. (2002). Light-emitting diode (LED) polymerization of dental composites: flexural properties and polymerization potential. *Biomater.* 1: 379–1385.

**33** Ak, A.T., Alpoz, A.R., Bayraktar, O., and Ertugrul, F. (2010). Monomer release from resin based dental materials cured with LED and halogen lights. *Eur. J. Dent.* 4: 34–40.

**34** Moraes, L.G., Rocha, R.S., Menegazzo, L.M. et al. (2008). Infrared spectroscopy: a tool for determination of the degree of conversion in dental composites. *J. Appl. Oral Sci.* 16: 145–149.

**35** Goldstein, R.E., Lamba, S., Lawson, N.C. et al. (2017). Microleakage around Class V composite restorations after ultrasonic scaling and sonic toothbrushing around their margin. *J. Esthet. Restor. Dent.* 29: 41–48.

**36** Mirzakhani, M., Mousavinasab, S.M., and Atai, M. (2016). The effect of acrylate-based dental adhesive solvent content on microleakage in composite restorations. *Dent. Res. J. (Isfahan)* 13: 515–520.

**37** Arends, J., Veen, H.v.d., Groeningen, G.v., and Schuthof, J. (2007). Quantified marginal leakage of composites in vitro. *J. Oral Rehabil.* 12 (3): 229–234.

**38** Moradi, S., Lomee, M., and Gharechahi, M. (2015). Comparison of fluid filtration and bacterial leakage techniques for evaluation of microleakage in endodontics. *Dent. Res. J. (Isfahan).* 12 (2): 109–114.

**39** Meyer, J.-M., Dennison, J., and Craig, R.G. (1974). Improved method of neutron activation analysis for microleakage studies. *J. Dent. Res.* 53: 356–363.

**40** Kang, Y.H., Shin, S.I., and Shin, D.H. (2004). A quantitative analysis about microleakage of all-in-one adhesives. *J. Korean Acad. Conserv. Dent.* 29 (1): 66–72.

**41** Mortensen DW, Boucher NE, Ryge G. A method of testing for marginal leakage of dental restorations with bacteria. J Dent Res 1965;44(1):58–63.

**42** Jokstad, A. (2016). Secondary caries and microleakage. *Dent. Mater.* 32 (1): 11–25.

**43** Marquezan, M., Corrêa, F.N., Sanabe, M.E. et al. (2009). Artificial methods of dentine caries induction: a hardness and morphological comparative study. *Arch. Oral. Biol.* 54: 1111–1117.

**44** Hembree, J.H. Jr. (1989). Microleakage at the gingival margin of Class II composite restorations with glass-ionomer liner. *J. Prosthet. Dent.* 61: 28–30.

**45** Fitchie, J.G., Reeves, G.W., Scarbrough, A.R., and Hembree, J.H. (1990). Microleakage of two new dentinal bonding systems. *Quintessence Int.* 21: 749–752.

**46** Going, R.E., Massler, M., and Dute, H.L. (1960). Marginal penetration of dental restorations by different radioactive isotopes. *J. Dent. Res.* 39: 273–284.

**47** Korntield B. (1953) Study of clinical behaviour of resins in operative dentistry. J. Dent. Res. 32, (abstr. 208), 714–715.

**48** Fernando de Goes, M. and Montes, M.A. (2004). Evaluation of silver methenamine method for nanoleakage. *J. Dent.* 32: 391–398.

**49** Costa, J.F., Siqueira, W.L., Loguercio, A.D. et al. (2011). Characterization of aqueous silver nitrate solutions for leakage tests. *J. Appl. Oral Sci.* 19: 254–259.

**50** Tomes, C.: paper to Odontological Society of Great Britain. British Journal o f Dental Science, 1875; 18: 239–240.

**51** Yavuz, I., Tumen, E.C., Kaya, C.A. et al. (2013). The reliability of microleakage studies using dog and bovine primary teeth instead of human primary teeth. *Eur. J. Paediatr. Dent.* 14: 42–46.

**52** Subramaniam, P. and Pandey, A. (2016). Assessment of microleakage of a composite resin restoration in primary teeth following Class III cavity preparation using Er, Cr: YSGG laser: an in vitro study. *J. Lasers Med. Sci.* 7: 172–176.

**53** Orłowski, M., Tarczydło, B., and Chałas, R. (2015). Evaluation of marginal integrity of four bulk-fill dental composite materials: in vitro study. *Sci. World J.* 2015: 701262.

**54** Fusayama, T. and Terachima, S. (1972). Differentiation of two layers of carious dentin by staining. *J. Dent. Res.* 51: 866.

**55** Raskin, A., Tassery, H., D'Hoore, W. et al. (2003). Influence of the number of sections on reliability of in vitro microleakage evaluations. *Am. J. Dent.* 16: 207–210.

**56** Kataia, E. and Kataia, M. (2016). Dye extraction method evaluation of the sealing ability of three types of endodontic sealers. *Egypt. Dent. J.* 62: 251–256.

**57** Gupta, A., Tavane, P., Gupta, P.K. et al. (2017). Evaluation of microleakage with total etch, self etch and universal adhesive systems in Class V restorations: an in vitro study. *J. Clin. Diagn. Res.* 11: ZC53-6.

**58** Jardine, A.P., Rosa, R.A., Santini, M.F. et al. (2016). The effect of final irrigation on the penetrability of an epoxy resin-based sealer into dentinal tubules: a confocal microscopy study. *Clin. Oral Investig.* 20: 117–123.

**59** Tangsgoolwatana, J., Cochran, M.A., Moore, B.K., and Li, Y. (1997). Microleakage evaluation of bonded amalgam restorations: confocal microscopy versus radioisotope. *Quintessence Int.* 28: 467–477.

**60** Swain, M.V. and Xue, J. (2009). State of the art of micro-CT applications in dental research. *Int. J. Oral Sci.* 1: 177–188.

**61** Carrera, C.A., Lan, C., Escobar-Sanabria, D. et al. (2015). The use of micro-CT with image segmentation to quantify leakage in dental restorations. *Dent. Mater.* 31: 382–390.

**62** Zavattini, A., Mancini, M., Higginson, J. et al. (2018). Micro-computed tomography evaluation of microleakage of Class II composite restorations: an in vitro study. *Eur. J. Dent.* 12 (3): 369–374.

**63** Mitropoulos, P., Rahiotis, C., Stamatakis, H., and Kakaboura, A. (2010). Diagnostic performance of the visual caries classification system ICDAS II versus radiography and micro-computed tomography for proximal caries detection: an *in vitro* study. *J. Dent.* 38: 859–867.

**64** Jia, S., Chen, D., Wang, D. et al. (2017). Comparing marginal microleakage of three different dental materials in veneer restoration using a stereomicroscope: an in vitro study. *BDJ Open* 3: 16010.

**65** Park, J.Y., Chung, J.H., Lee, J.S. et al. (2017). Comparisons of the diagnostic accuracies of optical coherence tomography, micro-computed tomography, and histology in periodontal disease: an ex vivo; study. *J. Periodontal Implant Sci.* 47: 30–40.

**66** Burghardt, A.J., Pialat, J.B., Kazakia, G.J. et al. (2013). Multicenter precision of cortical and trabecular bone quality measures assessed by high-resolution peripheral quantitative computed tomography. *J. Bone Miner Res.* 28: 524–536.

**67** Özkan, G., Kanli, A., Başeren, N.M., and Arslan, U. (2015). Tatar İ. Validation of micro-computed tomography for occlusal caries detection: an in vitro study. *Braz. Oral Res.* 29: S1806-83242015000100309.

**68** Yoshimine, N., Shimada, Y., Tagami, J., and Sadr, A. (2015). Interfacial adaptation of composite restorations before and after light curing: effects of adhesive and filling technique. *J. Adhes. Dent.* 17 (4): 329–336. https://doi.org/10.3290/j.jad.a34554.

**69** Lindberg, A., Van Dijken, J., and Hörstedt, P. (2005, 2005). in vivo interfacial adaptation of class II resin composite restorations with and without a flowable resin composite liner. *Clin. Oral Investig.* 9: 77–83.

**70** Muradov, M.A., Ryahovsky, A.N., Sorokina, D.R. et al. (2019). Study of the film thickness of dental composite resins after preheating. *Stomatologiya* 7, 98: 96.

**71** Ergücü, Z., Türkün, L.S., Onem, E., and Güneri, P. (2010). Comparative radiopacity of six flowable resin composites. *Oper. Dent.* 35: 436–440.

**72** Turgut, M.D., Attar, N., and Onen, A. (2003). Radiopacity of direct esthetic restorative materials. *Oper. Dent.* 28: 508–514.

# 3

# Isolation and Identification of Oral Microflora

**KEY CONCEPTS**

- Insight into the microflora of the oral cavity.
- Ability to design a microbiological study.
- Knowledge of the collection of different types of samples from the oral cavity, storage and transport prior to testing.
- The different methods of suspension and dilution, inoculation and incubation and identification of microorganisms.
- Understanding of the molecular biological methods and their working principle for the identification of microorganisms.

The human oral cavity contains a number of different habitats, including the teeth, gingival sulcus, tongue, hard and soft palates, and tonsils and provides appropriate space for the colonization of microorganisms. The microorganisms found in the human oral cavity have been referred to as the oral microflora, oral microbiota, or oral microbiome. Researchers have begun by identifying and characterizing the microorganisms with the largest representation within the communities of healthy mouths: *Streptococcus, Actinomyces, Veillonella, Fusobacterium, Porphromonas, Prevotella, Treponema, Nisseria, Haemophilis, Eubacteria, Lactobacterium, Capnocytophaga, Eikenella, Leptotrichia, Peptostreptococcus, Staphylococcus*, and *Propionibacterium* [1].

Under normal, "healthy" conditions, most of these microorganisms exist in our oral cavity in a symbiotic capacity, maintaining relationships with the host that are based on mutual benefits. The host receives the appropriate inflammatory stimulus from these commensal bacteria to maintain an effective but nondestructive inflammatory barrier against potential pathogens [1]. Also the commensal populations may keep pathogenic species in check by not allowing them to adhere to mucosal surfaces. As it changes from a commensal form to a pathogenic form, a microbial community may induce significant changes in tissue structure, with a breakdown of oral homeostasis [2].

*Manual of Laboratory Testing Methods for Dental Restorative Materials*, First Edition.
Paromita Mazumdar and Deepshikha Chowdhury.

Companion website: www.wiley.com/go/mazumdar/dental-restorative-materials

Approximately 700 prokaryote species that are present in the human oral cavity and 51% of which are officially named, 13% of which are not named (but cultivated) and 28% of which are known only as uncultivated phylotypes [3].

The microorganisms may colonize individually or form complex biofilms. The common diseases produced by oral microflora are dental caries, periodontitis, mucosal diseases, and oral cancer. The microorganisms causing dental caries and gingival diseases will be dealt with.

## 3.1 Isolation and Identification

The microorganisms are first isolated in order to be identified. Isolation is done by separating a strain from a mixed population of living microbes so that the microorganism of interest can be identified.

Since microorganisms in the oral cavity consist of a diverse population and there are new species being discovered very frequently, it is difficult to isolate and identify all the species. Moreover, most strains are nonpathogenic.

Phenotypic identification, i.e. cell morphology characteristics, is the basis for the identification of most microflora. This is the classical method for microbial identification. It constitutes observation of the phenotypic characteristics of a pure bacterial culture, including characteristic colonies (size, color, shape, etc.), cell characteristics (size, shape, arrangement, and stain), special structures (with or without spores, capsule, pili, and flagellum), culture characteristics (sensitivity to oxygen, optimum growth temperature, pH, requirements for nutrients and growth factors, etc.), metabolites, etc. [4].

Microbial culture has been used as the conventional technique for the identification of microorganisms, but recently advancements in research have led to the use of molecular techniques for more specific microflora identification [5]. Molecular biology involves evaluation of deoxyribonucleic acid (DNA), ribonucleic acid (RNA), and proteins thus having higher specificity and sensitivity over culture methods.

## 3.2 Steps for Conducting an Experiment for Microbial Isolation and Identification

The following steps are usually done for conducting an experiment.

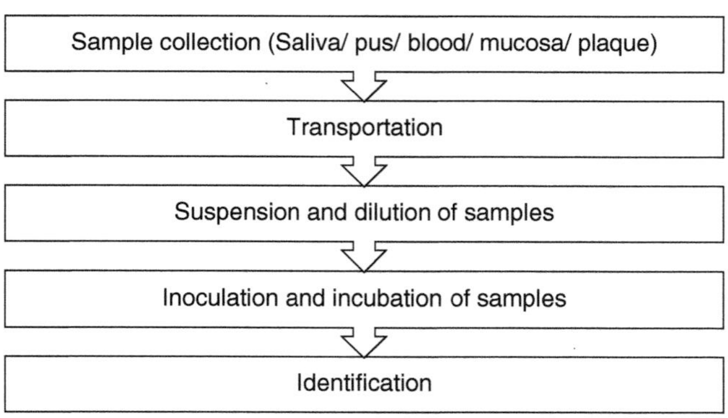

### 3.2.1 Sample Collection

Saliva and plaque samples are to analyze the prevalent microorganism as a contributing factor to dental caries. Infected tissue collection is done in order to analyze the pathogenic microorganism present in it to establish a diagnosis.

**Collection of saliva samples**: Saliva samples consist of stimulated salivary and unstimulated salivary samples. Stimulated salivary samples are collected when subjects are chewing paraffin or a rubber block, while unstimulated salivary samples are secreted naturally by the subjects. The best time for collection is early in the morning upon waking and before the teeth are brushed, or alternatively, samples can be collected between meals. Subjects should gently rinse their mouths with warm water to remove any food residue. About 0.5 to 1 ml of naturally secreted saliva is collected into a sample tube, or saliva samples can be directly taken from the oral cavity using sterile pipette tips [6].

**Things to Remember**

pH of unstimulated saliva ranges between 5.7 and 6.2, while the pH of stimulated saliva can reach 8. The flow rate of unstimulated saliva is 0.3–0.5 ml/min while that of stimulated saliva is 1–2 ml/min.

**Good to Know**

As dental plaque is not easily visible to the naked eye, its removal is difficult and complex. In order to remove dental plaque and improve the oral hygiene, the use of disclosing agents (dyes such as erythrosine, basic fuchsin, merbromin, fast green, etc.) has been recommended.

**Collection of plaque samples**: Plaque samples can be found on adjacent surfaces and fissures in occlusal surfaces. Before sample collection, subjects should gargle with warm water to remove any food residue. Then, sterile gauze or a yarn ball should be used to absorb saliva while plaque samples are collected. A sterile probe is commonly used in plaque collection from occlusal surface fissures. Plaque found on adjacent surfaces can be collected with sterile probe, dental floss, or fine orthodontic wire. Sterile curettes can be used to collect root surface plaque samples. Plaque samples on the gum or in the gingival margin can be collected using a spoon scaler [7].

**Collection of samples from infected tissues**: Samples of purulent fluid from a periodontal abscess can be collected with sterile syringes. Tissues in the alveolar socket are generally collected as samples of dry socket developed after tooth extraction [7].

### 3.2.2 Transportation of Samples for Testing

Fungal species, aerobic bacteria, and general facultative anaerobic bacteria can be collected by sterile cotton swab sampling and transported in sterile tubes available freely. For most anaerobic bacteria or microaerophilic bacteria, samples must be sent to the laboratory as soon as possible and maintained in an anaerobic environment. Pus or saliva samples that can be inserted directly into the sterile rubber stopper of the syringe needle used to collect the sample for transportation, most anaerobic samples must be placed in prereduced culture media and for transportation to the laboratory immediately after acquisition. This is to minimize the death of oxygen-sensitive bacteria during transportation [8].

For clinical specimens that cannot be examined in a timely manner or that must be transported over a long distance, anaerobic bags (commercially available) or prereduced liquid medium in a spiral tube sealed with liquid paraffin can be used for transportation [8].

**Good to Know**

When preparing pre-reduced media, one wants to:

1) drive off oxygen and partially reduce the ingredients by boiling,
2) then further reduce with cysteine, and
3) keep the medium oxygen free thereafter by flushing with oxygen-free gas and storing in tightly stoppered tubes (or bottles) containing oxygen-free gas.

In case if laboratory facility is not available immediately, then storage of the collected specimens is recommended. The guidelines given by International Agency for Research on Cancer (IARC) are as follows (Table 3.1).

**Table 3.1** Guidelines for storage of each specimen [8].

| Temperature in °C | Preservation method | Recommended for |
|---|---|---|
| +18 to +20 | Room temperature | Slides, tissue blocks |
| 0 to +4 | Refrigerator | Processing fresh specimens |
| −0.5 to −27 | Freezer | Short-term DNA stability |
| −27 to −40 | Freezer | DNA stability |
| −40 to −80 | Freezer | DNA/RNA stability |
| −30 to −130 | Freezer | Recommended for urine, blood, blood fractions (plasma, serum, etc.) |
| −130 to −150 | Liquid nitrogen vapor | Recommended for storage of tissues, preservation of cellular viability |
| −196 | Liquid nitrogen liquid phase | Storage of living cells |

*Source:* Miller [8].

### 3.2.3 Suspension and Dilution of Samples

In order to obtain pure cultures of individual bacteria, suspension of the samples is required prior to dilution. Proper dilution with the correct diluent must be performed prior to inoculation to obtain single colonies after sample suspension.

**Sample suspension**: There are two methods for sample suspension: spiral vortex oscillation and ultrasonic dispersion technique. Spiral vortex is easy to operate and has lower cost than the ultrasonic technique. The sample collection tube is placed on the vortex generator for 10–20 seconds. The oscillation creates a suspension. Ultrasonic dispersion produces a more uniform sample suspension. However, the equipment is expensive and some of the microorganisms can undergo lysis [9] (as shown in Figures 3.1 and 3.2).

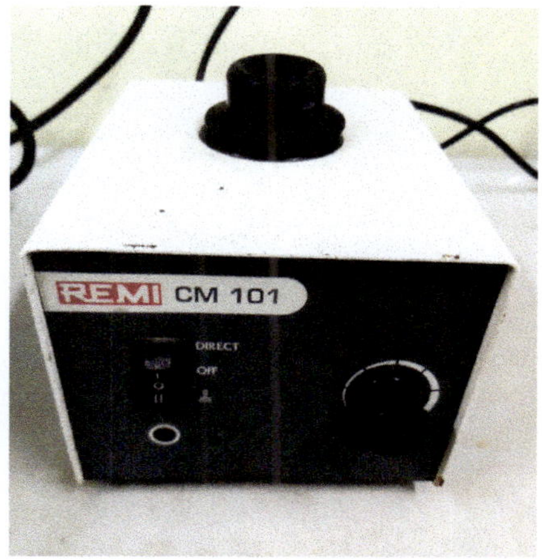


**Figure 3.1** Spin vortex.

**Sample dilution**: The solution in which the sample was transported can be used as a diluent, otherwise, phosphate buffer (pH 7.2) can also be used. A 10-fold dilution series is generally performed. Under aseptic conditions, 0.1 ml of the specimen sample is added to 0.9 ml diluents. After thorough mixing, 0.1 ml of the mixture (10−1) is added to a tube containing 0.9 ml diluent and mixed again. Using this method, 10-fold dilutions are made in series [9].

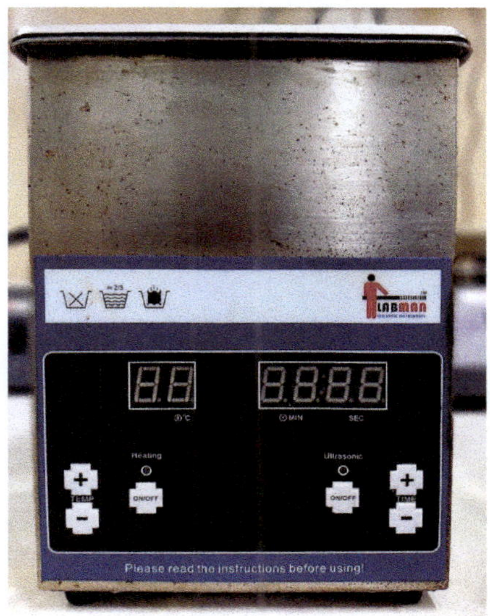


**Figure 3.2** Ultrasonic disperser.

### 3.2.4 Inoculation and Incubation of Samples

**Inoculation** is the process of introducing a sample directly into a flask or tube or spreading the sample on a culture medium. **Incubation** is the process of promoting growth of a culture on/in a media to increase the number for better identification. Incubation is done in an incubator [10]. (as shown in Figure 3.3).

**Inoculation of samples**: The media that are commonly used are brain-heart infusion (BHI) medium, trypticase soy medium (TSA), and trypticase phytone yeast extract (TPY) medium. For some obligate anaerobic gram-negative bacilli, 5% defibrinated blood (or 5% serum), chlorinated hemoglobin, and vitamin K1 must be supplied to the culture medium. To culture most aerobic and facultative anaerobic bacteria, the blood agar (BA) is used [10].

| Good to Know |
| --- |
| These media maybe prepared in the laboratory or maybe procured readymade from companies such as HiMedia, bioMérieux India. |

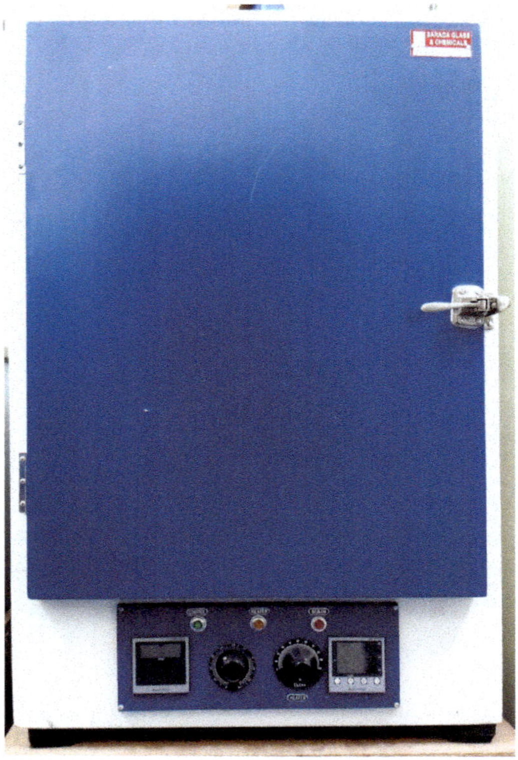

Figure 3.3 Incubator.

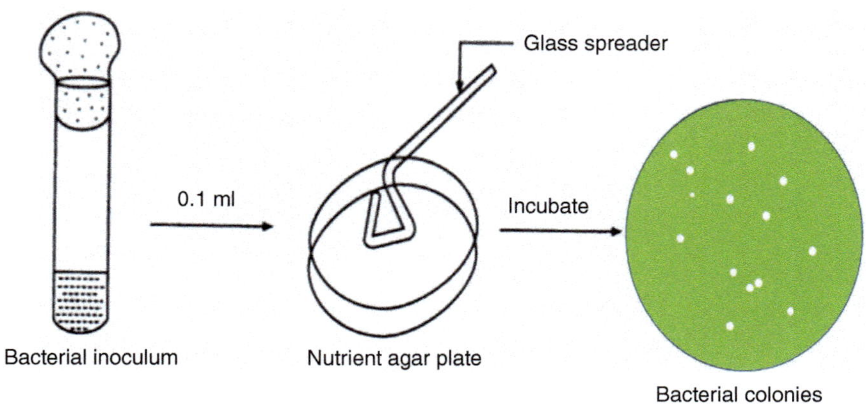


Figure 3.4 Spread method.

There are three commonly used methods for inoculation – the spread method, drop method and the spiral plate method [11].

a) **Spread method** – Ten microliters from appropriately diluted samples are taken with a micropipettor and placed on the surface of the agar medium. The sample is then evenly coated on the agar surface using a sterile glass spreader (triangle rod and L-shaped rod) (as shown in Figure 3.4).

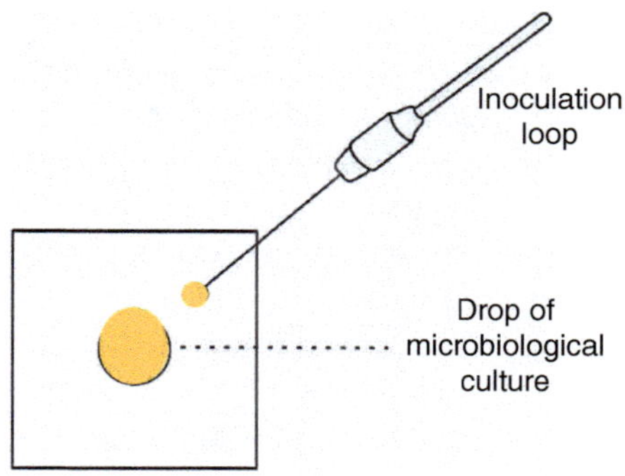


**Figure 3.5** Hanging drop method.

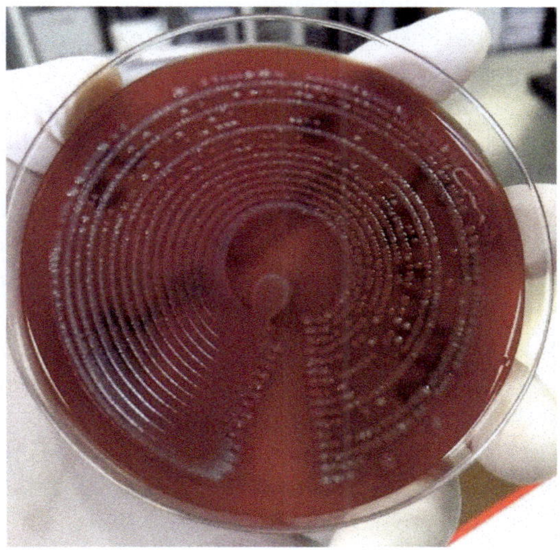

**Figure 3.6** Spiral plate method.

b) **Drop method** – Twenty-five or 50 μl samples at the appropriate dilution are dropped onto the surface of the agar using a micropipettor (as shown in Figure 3.5).
c) **Spiral plate method** – The sample liquid is automatically diluted and inoculated using a needle tip on the surface of the agar plate by the instrument, and the bacteria colonies grow uniformly along the spiral trajectory after incubation (as shown in Figure 3.6).

**Incubation of samples**: Some bacteria require incubation under the anaerobic conditions, while others require incubation under aerobic conditions. Anaerobic cultures grow best in atmospheric conditions with 80% $N_2$, 10% $CO_2$, and 10% $H_2$, with a temperature of 36–37 °C and approximately 48–72 hours culture time [10, 12]. Commonly used anaerobic incubation devices include the anaerobic glove box, anaerobic incubator, anaerobic bag, etc.

### 3.2.5 Identification of Microflora

The initial steps of bacterial identification involve observing colony morphology following incubation and performing Gram stain. The Gram stain helps us know whether the bacteria is gram positive or gram negative. It also tells us the shape of the microorganisms. After this, a second round of purification is carried out to further complete phenotypic and genotypic identification using routine protocols for microbial separation and identification. Bacterial colony morphology can be described in terms of its size, color, shape, and growth pattern. Various reports of Gram's stain sensitivity suggest a range from 50% to 90%. The specificity approaches 100% [13, 14].

The problem with gram staining lies in the fixation step. If bacteria is not fixed, the microorganisms will get washed out and the microscope will show a blank slide [15].

**Microscopes used for identification**: Optical microscope, Stereomicroscope, Scanning electron microscope, Confocal laser scanning microscope, and Transmission electron microscope. The magnification range of different microscopes has been mentioned in table 3.2.

Apart from the optical microscope, the remaining types provide high resolution and three-dimensional images thereby allowing better visibility and characterization of the morphology.

**Colony counting**: After inoculation and incubation of the microorganisms, viable bacteria form colonies that are viewed under the microscope. Colony counting maybe done manually or using automatic colony counting machines (as shown in Figure 3.7).

Manual colony counting is done by counting each colony dot once. The Petri dish is set on a grid background and the colonies in each grid cell are counted, moving in a methodical pattern through all of the cells. Marking counted colonies on the back of the Petri dish can also be a helpful approach [16].

Automated colony counters [16] take an image of the dish, separate out the colonies from the background and then use an algorithm to count the colonies on the plate, e.g. EasyCount 2 (bioMérieux India).

Nowadays, **biochemical tests** are carried out for their rapid identification. These tests kits are commercially available such as the HiIMViC (HiMedia) and Biochemical Test Kit I (Sisco). Microbial biochemistry tests shorten the time required to identify microbes, reduce costs, and ensure or enhance the accuracy of identification of an unknown sample. It is the fastest developing trend in microbial identification.

**Table 3.2** Magnification range of different microscopes.

| Microscope type | Magnification range |
|---|---|
| Optical microscope | 10× – ocular lens and 100× objective lens<br>Total magnification – 1000× |
| Stereomicroscope | 2× to 100× |
| Scanning electron microscope | 20×–30 000× |
| Transmission electron microscope | Total magnification is a combination of objective lens × magnification of intermediate lens × magnification of projector lens. Each of these is 100× |
| Confocal laser scanning microscope | 120× to 15 000× |

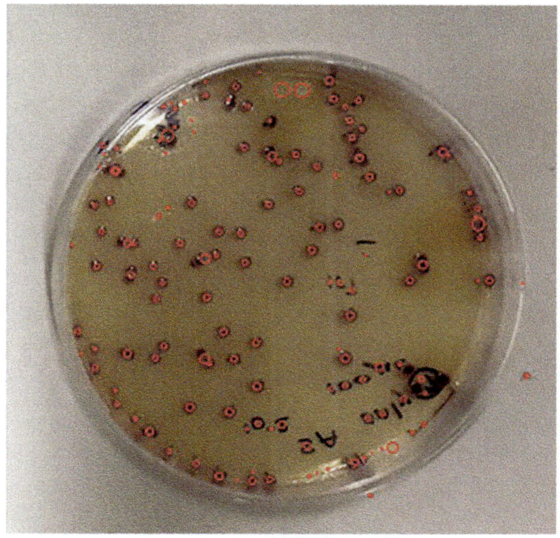

**Figure 3.7** Manual colony counting.

## 3.3 Molecular Biological Methods for Microflora Identification

The conventional culture techniques have distinctive advantages, but have limitations some of which include the need to preserve the bacterial viability, identification of low numbers of microorganisms, transport conditions, labor intensiveness, need expert personnel, elongated period of time before outcomes, and strict sampling.

The newer techniques of molecular biology involve evaluation of DNA, RNA, and proteins.

Molecular biology techniques have several advantages over the conventional culture methods which are as follows:

- Detection of both cultivable and uncultivable microbial species or strains.
- Higher specificity and accurate identification of microbial strains.
- Detection of microbial species directly in clinical samples, without the need for cultivation.
- Higher sensitivity.
- Less time consuming thus offering rapid diagnosis.
- They do not require carefully controlled anaerobic conditions during sampling and transportation, which is advantageous since fastidious anaerobic bacteria and other fragile microorganisms can lose viability during transit.
- A large number of samples can be stored and analyzed all at once.

The techniques that are commonly used are

1) Polymerase chain reaction (PCR) and its variants.
2) DNA–DNA hybridization.
3) Fluorescence in situ hybridization.
4) Terminal restriction fragment length polymorphism analysis (T-RFLP).
5) DNA microarrays.

### 3.3.1 Polymerase Chain Reaction

PCR method amplifies the genes and their RNA transcripts isolated from several sources such as saliva, gingival crevicular fluid, subgingival plaque, etc. Each PCR test needs the presence of DNA polymerase enzyme, extracted DNA sample, primers, and nucleotides.

**Template extracted DNA** is the identified target sequence that requires to be amplified.

**DNA polymerase** is a key enzyme to replicate target sequences of DNA that attaches individual nucleotides together to generate the PCR product.

**Primer molecules** are appropriate short and single-stranded sequences of DNA or RNA designed to particularly anneal to a desired nucleic acid target.

For PCR amplification, DNA is extracted from a desired target and added to the reaction mix tube including primers, PCR buffer, deoxynucleotides (dNTP), $MgCl_2$, and DNA polymerase enzyme in an examination tube.

The reaction tube then located in a thermocycler that runs repeated cycles of DNA replication that takes place in the following steps: [9]

1) **Denaturation of DNA**: The reaction tube is heated to 94 °C for separation of the double-stranded DNA and yielding two single strands of DNA molecules.
2) **Annealing**: At 50–65 °C, forward and reverse primers anneal to a particular site at each of the single-stranded DNA templates.
3) **Extension or elongation**: At 72 °C, new complementary DNA strands synthesizes by the elongation of primers using DNA polymerase enzyme (as shown in Figure 3.8).

To evaluate the amplified PCR product (Table 3.3) which the usual is to recognize the product by size after movement through **electrophoresis technique** on an agarose gel or polyacrylamide gel stained with SYBR Gold or SYBR Green or ethidium bromide (as shown in Figure 3.9).

| Things to Remember |
|---|
| It takes almost 30–40 cycles to get a result in a conventional PCR machine. |

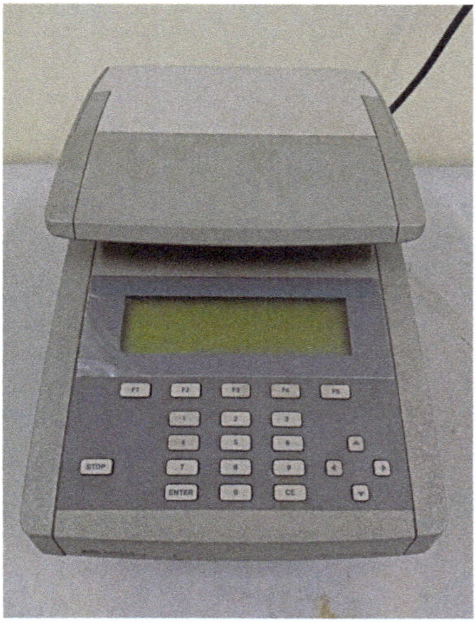


**Figure 3.8** Conventional PCR machine.

**Table 3.3** The different variants of the PCR [20–22].

| Types of PCR | Variation in method | Application |
|---|---|---|
| Hot start PCR | The polymerases used in Hot Start PCR are unreactive at ambient temperatures | Increases DNA product and specificity of PCR method by decreasing nonspecific product in the initial step of PCR reaction |
| Nested PCR | Two primer sets are used sequentially. The first set is applied to amplify a target sequence then the acquired amplicons is utilized as the target sequence for a second PCR reaction by internal primers | Reduce non-specific binding in products due to the amplification of unexpected primer binding sites |
| Allele-specific PCR | Primers have the SNP in 3′ ends that bind and match exactly to target DNA sequences | Detect the single-nucleotide polymorphisms (SNPs) at a particular location of genome |
| Multiplex PCR | Utilize multiple primer sets in a single PCR reaction to produce amplicons with different sizes | Capability to examination for different target genes and organisms by one PCR reaction |
| RAPD (Random Amplification of Polymorphic DNA) PCR | Use short arbitrary primers (8–12 nucleotides) to amplify fragments | Characterize and trace the phylogeny of animal species |
| Reverse transcription PCR (RT-PCR) | RNA molecule via a reverse transcriptase enzyme is converted into cDNA molecule and then utilized as template sequence | Detect RNA expression |
| Quantitative PCR (qPCR) or real-time PCR | Use of fluorophore-containing DNA probes, such as TaqMan or fluorescent dyes | Quantify the PCR product |
| Colony PCR | Bacterial colonies are screened directly by PCR | Screen for correct DNA vector constructs |
| Digital PCR (dPCR) | No need of reference standards | Evaluates the quantity of DNA or RNA molecules exists in a sample |
| Repetitive element sequence-based PCR (rep-PCR) | Utilizes oligonucleotide primers based on short repetitive sequence elements distributed all over the bacterial genome | General typing technique for DNA fingerprinting and discrimination of bacterial strains |
| Assembly PCR | Production of long DNA sequences on a pool of long sequences with short overlapping sequences, to assemble two or more fragments of DNA into one fragment | Amplification of interspersed repetitive DNA elements present at distinct locations in prokaryotic genomes |

*Source:* Farber [20], Abulreesh et al. [21], and Taponen et al. [22].

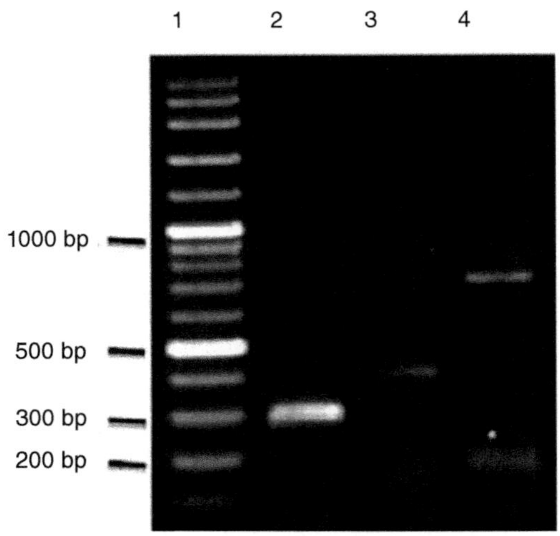


**Figure 3.9** Agarose gel electrophoresis.

### 3.3.2 DNA–DNA Hybridization

DNA hybridization is the process of joining two single strands of DNA thus forming dsDNA. Joining of the two strands is facilitated by the formation of hydrogen bonds between the nucleotide bases. DNA hybridization may be used to assess the genetic similarity between two populations of DNA or to detect a specific sequence of DNA in a population of DNA molecules. This is achieved by using a nucleic acid probe [17].

| **Things to Remember** |
|---|
| DNA hybridization methodology employs DNA probes that are single-stranded DNA, labeled with an enzyme, radioactive isotope or a chemiluminescence reporter that can locate and bind to their complementary nucleic acid sequences. |

During DNA hybridization, the hydrogen bonds of the target DNA are disrupted by incubating at 95 °C or exposure to an alkaline pH. This leads to the formation of ssDNA. The target ssDNA is incubated with the probe at approximately 65 °C or below for a prolonged period. If the target DNA sequence is complementary to the probe sequence, then hybridization will occur by the formation of hydrogen bonds. The greater the complementarity, the greater the stability of the bonds formed between the target and the probe [17] (as shown in Figure 3.10).

### 3.3.3 Fluorescence in Situ Hybridization

Fluorescence in situ hybridization (FISH) involves rRNA-targeted oligonucleotide probe. This technique detects nucleic acid sequences by a fluorescent labeled probe that hybridizes specifically to its complementary target sequence within the intact cell. In addition to

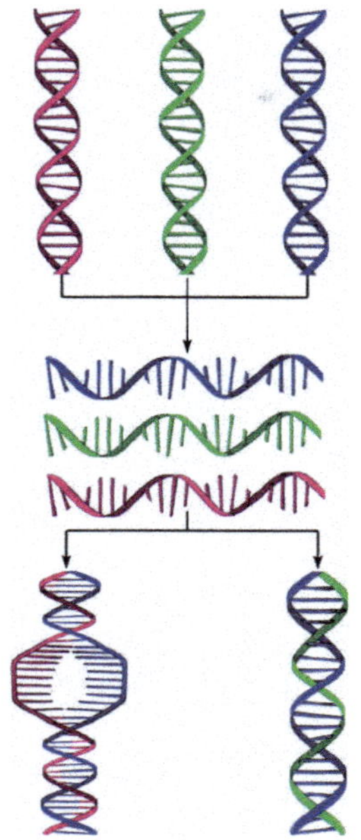


**Figure 3.10** Diagrammatic representation of DNA hybridization.

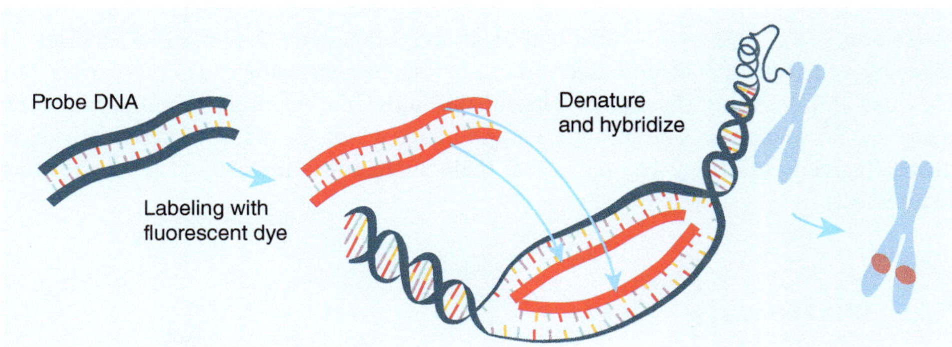


**Figure 3.11** Diagrammatic representation of Fluorescence in situ hybridization.

identification, FISH gives information about presence, morphology, number, organization, and spatial distribution of microorganisms [18]

A typical FISH protocol includes four steps:

- the fixation and permeabilization of the sample
- hybridization with the respective probes for detecting the respective target sequences
- washing steps to remove unbound probe
- detection of labeled cells by microscopy or flowcytometry (as shown in Figure 3.11).

### 3.3.4 Terminal-RFLP

T-RFLP is a recent molecular approach that can assess subtle genetic differences between microbial strains as well as provide insight into the structure and function of microbial communities. It is used for profiling of microbial communities based on the position of a

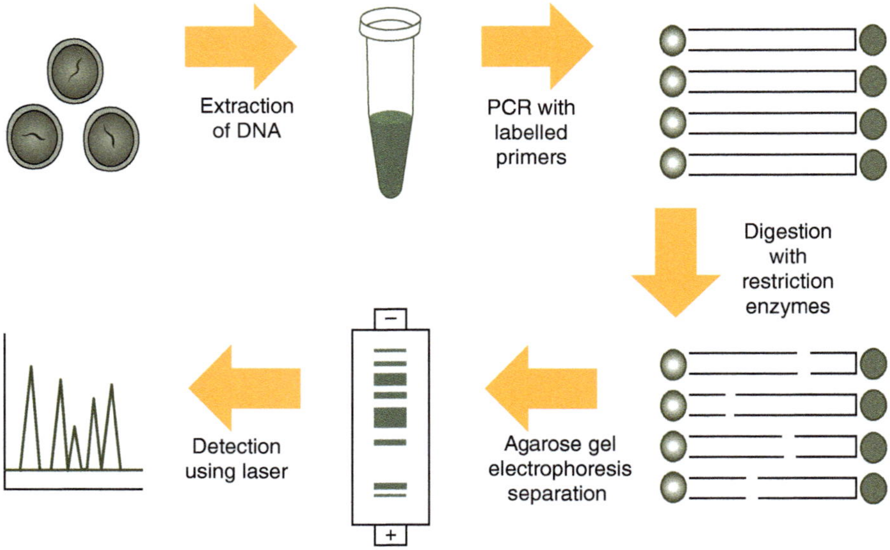


**Figure 3.12** Diagrammatic representation of T-RFLP. *Source:* Based on Krishnan et al. [12].

restriction site closest to a labeled end of an amplified gene. The method is based on digesting a mixture of PCR amplified variants of a single gene using one or more restriction enzymes and detecting the size of each of the individual resulting terminal fragments using a DNA sequencer. The result is a graph image where the *x*-axis represents the sizes of the fragment and the *y*-axis represents their fluorescence intensity [12] (as shown in Figure 3.12).

### 3.3.5 DNA Microarrays

DNA microarray methods were first described in 1995 and essentially consist of many probes that are discretely located on a nonporous solid support, such as a glass slide. After a PCR is used to amplify microbial DNA from clinical specimens, microarrays can then be used to identify the PCR products by hybridization to an array that is composed of species-specific probes. When coupled to PCR, microarrays have detection sensitivity similar to conventional molecular methods with the added ability to discriminate several species at a time [19] (as shown in Figure 3.13).

| **Good to Know** |
|---|
| Restriction Enzymes (endonucleases): molecular scissors that cut DNA.<br>Each enzymes has a microbial origin.<br>For example: *TaqI*: Thermus aquaticus YTI. |

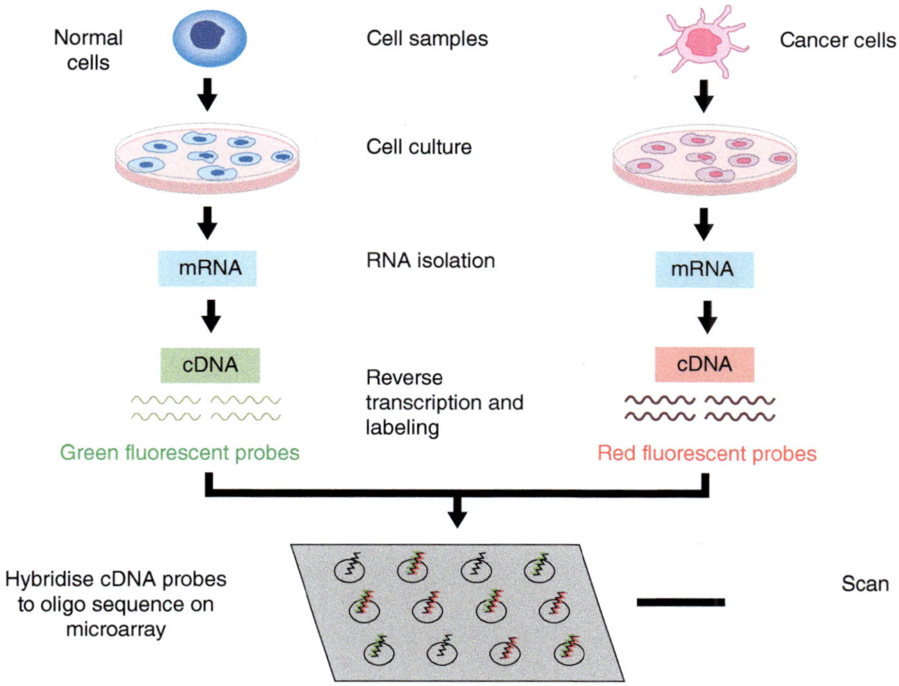


**Figure 3.13** Diagrammatic representation of DNA microarray. *Source:* Based on Parolin et al. [19].

This chapter will be beneficial for researchers while testing for oral microflora and their role in dental caries along with the antimicrobial efficacy of dental restorative materials. Isolation and identification of microorganisms have an important role in endodontics as well which is beyond the scope of this handbook.

**Key Points**

1) Microbial isolation is done by separating a strain from a mixed population of living microbes so that the microorganism of interest can be identified.
2) Microbial culture is the conventional technique for identification of microorganisms, but recently molecular techniques are used for more specific microflora identification.
3) Sample to be tested are collected followed by storage and transport to the laboratory for testing. In the laboratory, they are suspended and diluted followed by inoculation and incubation and finally identification of the microorganism.
4) Molecular biology involve evaluation of DNA, RNA, and proteins. They have high sensitivity and specificity.
5) The molecular biological techniques for identification involve PCR and its variants, DNA–DNA hybridization, fluorescence in situ hybridization, T-RFLP and DNA microarrays.

## References


1 Jenkinson, H.F. and Lamont, R.J. (2005). Oral microbial communities in sickness and in health. *Trends Microbiol.* 13 (12): 589–595.

2 Library LAN ed (2009). *Los Alamos National Library*. Livermore: ORALGEN.

3 Paster, B.J., Olsen, I., Aas, J.A., and Dewhirst, F.E. (2006). The breadth of bacterial diversity in the human periodontal pocket and other oral sites. *Periodontology 2000* 42: 80–87.

4 Rosselló-Mora, R. and Amann, R. (2001). The species concept for prokaryotes. *FEMS Microbiol. Rev.* 25 (1): 39–67.

5 Franco-Duarte, R., Černáková, L., Kadam, S. et al. (2019). Advances in chemical and biological methods to identify microorganisms-from past to present. *Microorganisms* 7 (5): 130.

6 Gomar-Vercher, S., Simón-Soro, A., Montiel-Company, J.M. et al. (2018). Stimulated and unstimulated saliva samples have significantly different bacterial profiles. *PLoS One* 13 (6): e0198021.

7 Xian, P., Xuedong, Z., Xin, X. et al. (2018). The oral microbiome bank of China. *Int. J. Oral Sci.* 10 (2): 16.

8 Miller, J.M. (1996). *A Guide to Specimen Management in Clinical. Microbiology*, 153. Washington. ISBN 1-55581-105-1: ASM Press.

9 Aas, J.A., Paster, B.J., Stokes, L.N. et al. (2005). Defining the normal bacterial flora of the oral cavity. *J. Clin. Microbiol.* 43: 5721–5732.

10 Pozhitkov, A.E., Beikler, T., Flemmig, T., and Noble, P.A. (2011). High-throughput methods for analysis of the human oral microbiome. *Periodontology 2000* 55: 70–86.

11 Jarvis, B., Lach, V., and Wood, J. (2008). Evaluation of the spiral plate maker for the enumeration of micro-organisms in foods. *J. Appl. Microbiol.* 43: 149–157.

12 Krishnan, K., Chen, T., and Paster, B.J. (2017). A practical guide to the oral microbiome and its relation to health and disease. *Oral Dis.* 23: 276–286.

13 Baron, E.J., Peterson, L.R., and Finegold, S.M. (eds.) (1994). *Bailey & Scott's Diagnostic Microbiology*, 9e, 69–70. St Louis, MO: Mosby.

14 McClelland, R. (2001). Gram's stain: the key to microbiology. *MLO Med. Lab. Obs.* 33: 20-2–25-8.

15 Kayser, F.H. (2005). Haemophilus and Pasteurella. In: *Medical Microbiology*, 10e (eds. H. Fritz, F.H. Kayser, A. Kurt, et al.), 300–301. Stuttgart: Georg Thieme Verlag.

16 Sanders, E.R. (2012). Aseptic laboratory techniques: plating methods. *J. Vis. Exp.* 63: e3064.

17 Socransky, S.S., Smith, C., Martin, L. et al. (1994). "Checkerboard" DNA–DNA hybridization. *BioTechniques* 17 (4): 788–792.

18 O'Connor, C. (2008). Fluorescence in situ hybridization (FISH). *Nat. Educ.* 1 (1): 171.

19 Parolin, C., Giordani, B., Palomino, R.A.Ñ. et al. (2017). Design and validation of a DNA-microarray for phylogenetic analysis of bacterial communities in different oral samples and dental implants. *Sci. Rep.* 7 (1): 6280.

20 Farber, J.M. (1996). An introduction to the hows and whys of molecular typing. *J. Food Prot.* 59: 1091–1101.

**21** Abulreesh, H.H., Paget, T.A., and Goulder, R. (2006). *Campylobacter* in waterfowl and aquatic environments: incidence and methods of detection. *Environ. Sci. Tech.* 40: 7122–7131.

**22** Taponen, S., Salmikivi, L., Simojoki, H. et al. (2009). Real-time polymerase chain reaction-based identification of bacteria in milk samples from bovine clinical mastitis with no growth in conventional culturing. *Dairy Sci.* 92 (6): 2610–2617.

# 4

# Assessment of Biocompatibility of Dental Materials

**KEY CONCEPTS**

- Knowledge of the different standards that regulate biocompatibility assessment.
- Understanding of the phases in which biocompatibility testing is carried out.
- A detailed understanding of the different types of cytotoxicity tests.
- Different types of animal tests such as inhalation test, implantation test, maximization test, Buehler's test.
- Understanding of the usage tests.
- The different phases of a clinical trial.
- Ability to differentiate between the phases of the biocompatibility testing.

The oral environment is complex owing to periodic changes in pH, temperature, different stress patterns, saliva, different food habits, and varied masticatory forces. Any material placed in the oral cavity is in direct contact with the tissues. It should not contain any toxic substance that can directly harm the dental and mucosal tissues or induce systemic effects by getting absorbed into the circulatory system. The material in the oral cavity must be compatible with the living tissue. Thus, all dental materials are subjected to biocompatibility testing prior to their commercial release. Biocompatibility has been defined as "the ability of a material to function in the presence of an appropriate host response." [1]. Biocompatibility of dental materials is characterized by many parameters such as toxicity, allergenicity, genotoxicity, mutagenicity, carcinogenicity, and teratogenicity. Thus, it is impossible to characterize a particular material by a single test method. A series of in vitro and in vivo tests are conducted for the assessment of biocompatibility of a dental material [2].

## 4.1 Standards for Testing Biocompatibility

In order to make the testing more uniform, the tests need to be standardized by regulatory bodies. The American National Standards Institute/American Dental Association (ANSI/ADA) 41 and the ISO 10993 and ISO 7405 are the standards for the testing of biocompatibility of dental materials [3].

*Manual of Laboratory Testing Methods for Dental Restorative Materials*, First Edition.
Paromita Mazumdar and Deepshikha Chowdhury.

Companion website: www.wiley.com/go/mazumdar/dental-restorative-materials

ISO 10993-12 standard describes the types of test samples, suitable extraction vehicles and conditions, and appropriate reference materials to be used as controls (Table 4.1). The standard recommends testing materials in their final product form and condition whenever possible. If finished materials are not available for testing, the evaluation of representative subcomponents is acceptable in some cases. As the last option, representative samples of the formulated materials that have been preconditioned by the same processing steps as the final product should be tested. If the material is too large or cannot be tested as a whole for some other reason, each individual material having the potential of coming in contact with body tissues should be represented in the same proportion in the test sample as it is in the final product. In all cases, the standard requires that the samples be handled in such a manner as to avoid contamination [4].

### 4.1.1 ANSI/ADA 41

The tests are divided into initial, secondary and usage tests and follows the linear progression test program (Autian 1970) [1] (Table 4.2).

### 4.1.2 ISO 10993

The document divides the tests into initial, supplementary and specialized tests [4] (Table 4.3).

**Table 4.1** Suitable extraction ratios for test materials of various thicknesses.

| Thickness (mm) | Extraction ratio[a] ±10% | Examples of material |
|---|---|---|
| ≤0.5 | 6 $cm^2$/ml | Metal, synthetic polymer, ceramic, composite film, sheet, and tubing walls |
| >0.5 | 3 $cm^2$/ml | Metal, synthetic polymer, ceramic, composite tubing walls, slab, and molded items |
| ≤1.0 | 3 $cm^2$/ml | Natural elastomer |
| >1.0 | 1.25 $cm^2$/ml | Natural elastomer |
| Irregular | 0.1–0.2 g/ml, 6 $cm^2$/ml | Pellets |

[a] The ratio of the surface area or mass of the test sample to the volume of extractant used.

**Table 4.2** ANSI/ADA 41 biocompatibility tests for dental materials.

| Initial tests | In vitro tests for cytotoxicity, membrane analysis, mutagenicity and carcinogenicity, and animal tests for systemic toxicity |
|---|---|
| Animal tests | Animal tests for inflammatory and immune response |
| Usage tests | Tests for pulpal and bone response |

**Table 4.3** ISO 10993 biocompatibility tests for dental materials.

| **Initial tests** | **In vitro and animal tests for cytotoxicity, sensitization and systemic toxicity** |
|---|---|
| Supplementary tests | Tests for chronic toxicity, carcinogenicity, and biodegradation. These tests can be carried out on both humans and animals |
| Specialized tests | Dentin barrier test |

### 4.1.3 ISO 7405

This document includes the preclinical evaluation of biocompatibility of medical devices used in dentistry. It includes the usage tests such as pulp–dentin tests and pulp capping/pulpotomy tests [4].

## 4.2 Testing Hierarchy

The biocompatibility tests are divided into three basic phases: [1–4]

1) **Primary phase** – initial in vitro tests
2) **Secondary phase** – involves animal tests
3) **Usage phase** – involves tests in a clinical situation or set-up.

The testing may be done in two ways – linear progression or nonlinear progression.

### 4.2.1 Linear Progression

Autian in 1970 had developed this pattern of testing in accordance with the cumulative measure of biocompatibility. It was a linear paradigm from primary through usage tests where the material has to clear the previous tests to be eligible for the next test (as shown in Figure 4.1).

**Limitation**: In vitro and animal studies do not accurately predict the results of the usage tests. For example, at cellular level, zinc oxide eugenol is cytotoxic; however in a clinical scenario, it has mild irritating effects on the pulp and is used for pulp capping.

### 4.2.2 Nonlinear Progression

Mjör et al. compared in vitro, animal and usage tests for clinical usage and found the materials that cleared the first two tests were not entirely harmless at the clinical usage level. Thus, in 1977, he modified the linear paradigm to a nonlinear pattern, where simultaneously all three tests would be performed on the tested material.

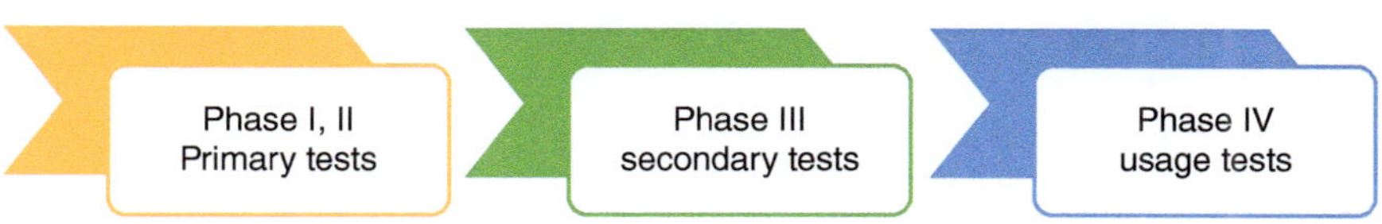


**Figure 4.1** Linear progression of testing hierarchy.

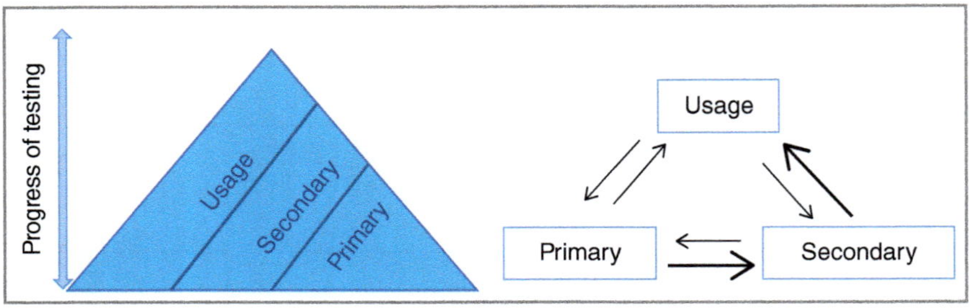


**Figure 4.2** Nonlinear progression of testing hierarchy.

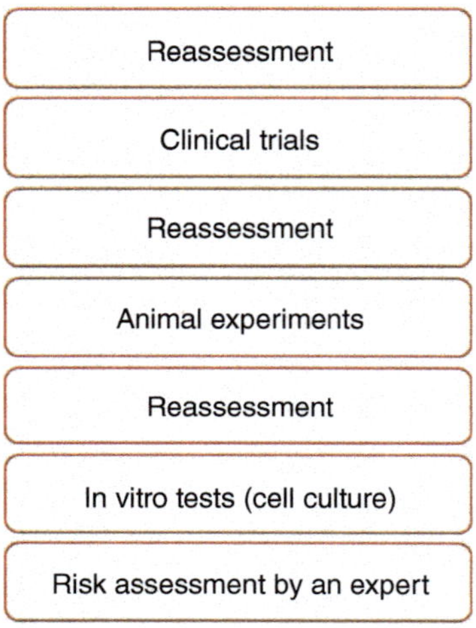


**Figure 4.3** Biocompatibility testing based on risk assessment (US-FDA 2016).

All the tests are initially conducted simultaneously but as the testing progresses, the usage tests predominate (as shown in Figure 4.2).

Currently, the choice of test method is based on the risk assessment. The risk assessment is the basis of deciding whether new tests are necessary or not (as shown in Figure 4.3).

## 4.3 Initial Tests for Assessment of Biocompatibility

Prior to animal and human testing, a material has to undergo a series of in vitro or laboratory test. The recommended testing methods include

For in vitro cytotoxicity screening, the different testing methods include [5, 6]

Direct cell culture test:

i) Barrier screening test
ii) Agar diffusion testing
iii) Filter diffusion testing
iv) Tooth slice culture assay
v) Micronuclei test

vi) Ame's test
vii) Style's test
viii) Hemolysis test

### 4.3.1 Direct Cell Culture Test

**Good to Know**

Primary cell culture – these are normal cells freshly taken from the body and cultured. They are capable of only limited growth in culture.

Continuous cell lines – these are cells of single type, usually derived from cancer cells, that are capable of continuous serial cultivation indefinitely. These are primary cells that have been transformed previously to allow them to grow more or less indefinitely in culture.

Primary cell cultures are more relevant than continuous cell lines for measuring cytotoxicity of materials.

Animal or human tissues (mouse fibroblasts [L-929, 3T3] or human epithelial cells [HeLa]) are used for these tests after growing them under suitable conditions on culture plates. Each type of tissue requires specific conditions for reproduction. Isolation of these cells can be done in a laboratory or they can be purchased from ATCC. The cells are kept in until a monolayer of cells is obtained. The material to be tested is then added to the culture and allowed to be in contact for 72 hours. Changes in the characteristics of the cell lines are observed under the microscope. Often, dyes are used to analyze cell damage. The vital cells take up the stain in contrast to the cells exhibiting membrane rupture [7].

One of the innate disadvantages of these cell counts is the inability to distinguish between living and dead cells if no morphological alterations have occurred. The viable cell count can be extremely subjective, and any artifact further compounds the problem [7].

There are several types of direct cell culture tests based on their principle of testing. These are as follows:

i) **Dye exclusion**: Trypan blue, eosin, Congo red, erythrosine B assays.
ii) **Colorimetric assays**: MTT assay, MTS assay, XTT assay, WST-1 assay, WST-8 assay, lactate dehydrogenase (LDH) assay, sulforhodamine B (SRB) assay, neutral red uptake (NRU) assay, and crystal violet assay (CVS).
iii) **Fluorometric assays**: alamarBlue (AB) assay and CFDA-AM assay.
iv) **Luminometric assays**: adenosine tri-phosphate (ATP) assay and real-time viability assay.

#### 4.3.1.1 Dye Exclusion Assays

The simplest and widely used is the dye exclusion method. In dye exclusion method, only the viable cells exclude dyes and become colorless, but dead cells are unable to exclude them. A variety of dyes including eosin, Congo red, erythrosine B, and trypan blue are used. Amongst these, trypan blue is commonly used [8].

If dye exclusion assays are used, following factors must be considered:

i) lethally damaged cells by cytotoxic agents may require several days to lose their membrane integrity,
ii) the surviving cells may continue to proliferate during this time, and
iii) some of the lethally damaged cells may lose their membrane integrity at an early stage causing dye uptake thus giving false results.

Dye exclusion assays are comparatively simple, require small numbers of cells, are rapid, and are capable of detecting cell viability accurately in nondividing cell populations.

**Disadvantages**: The technique cannot distinguish between healthy cells and damaged viable cells. Cell counting is generally done using a hemocytometer. Therefore, counting errors can occur due to poor dispersion of cells, cell loss during cell dispersion, inaccurate dilution of cells, improper filling of the chamber and presence of air bubbles in the chamber.

#### 4.3.1.2 Colorimetric Assays

It measures a biochemical marker to evaluate metabolic activity of the cells. Reagents used in colorimetric assays develop a color in response to the cell viability, allowing the colorimetric measurement of cell viability via spectrophotometer. Colorimetric assays are applicable for adherent or suspended cell lines. They are easy to perform, and comparably economical. Commercial kits of colorimetric assays are available from companies such as Thermofisher, Sigma Aldrich.

***MTT Assay*** MTT (3-(4,5-dimethylthiazol-2-yl)-2–5-diphenyltetrazolium bromide) assay is one of the most commonly used colorimeteric assay to assess cytotoxicity or cell viability. It was developed by Mossman in 1980. It is also known as Mossman's Tetrazoleum Assay. This assay determines cell viability by measuring activity of the enzyme succinate dehydrogenase present in the mitochondria. In this assay, MTT (yellow color) is reduced to a purple colored formazan by NADH (nicotinamide adenine dinucleotide + hydrogen). This product can be quantified by light absorbance at a specific wavelength [9–11].

**Advantages**: This method is easy to use, is safe, has a high reproducibility and is widely used to determine cell viability.

**Disadvantages**: MTT formazan is insoluble in water, and it forms purple needle-shaped crystals in the cells. Therefore, prior to measuring the absorbance, an organic solvent such as dimethyl sulfoxide (DMSO) or isopropanol is required to solubilize the crystals. Additionally, the cytotoxicity of MTT formazan makes it difficult to remove cell culture media from the plate wells due to floating cells with MTT formazan needles, giving significant well-to-well error (as shown in Figure 4.4).

***MTS Assay*** The MTS assay (5-(3-carboxymethoxyphenyl)-2-(4,5-dimethyl-thiazoly)-3-(4-sulfophenyl) tetrazolium, inner salt assay) is a colorimetric assay. This assay is based on the same principle as the MTT assay discussed above [12, 13].

**Advantages**: This assay provides ideal properties for cytotoxicity measurement because it is easy to use, rapid, reliable, and inexpensive. Therefore, it can be used for onsite toxicological assessments.

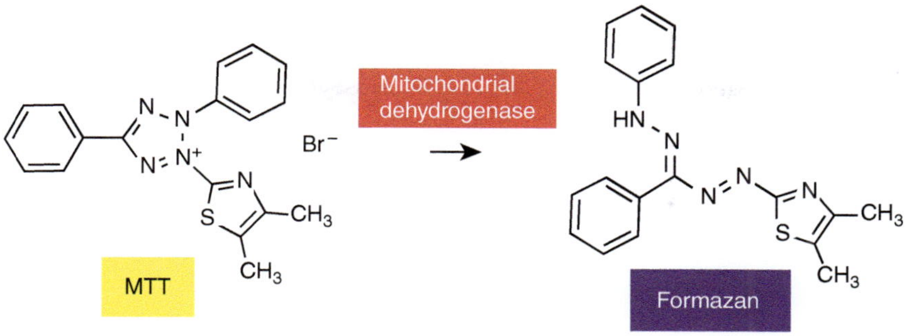


**Figure 4.4** MTT assay.

**Table 4.4** In vitro tests for commonly used dental materials.

| Test | Materials |
|---|---|
| Direct cell culture test | Noble metals and base metals, alloys, ceramics, silver amalgam, adhesive resins, gypsum products, and impression materials |
| Barrier screening test | Dental cements including bioceramic cements |
| Agar diffusion testing | Dental cements including bioceramic cements and alloys |
| Filter diffusion testing | Noble metals and base metals, alloys, ceramics, silver amalgam, and dental cements |
| Tooth slice culture assay | Composite resin |
| Micronuclei test | Genotoxicity testing of dental materials |
| Ame's test and Style's test | Mutagenicity of dental materials |
| Hemolysis test | Alloys |

**Disadvantages**: The level of absorbance measured at 492 nm is influenced by the incubation time, cell type, and cell number. The proportion of MTS detection reagents to cells in culture also influences the measured absorbance level. Previous studies suggested a linear relationship between incubation time and absorbance for short incubation times up to five hours. Therefore, proper incubation time for this assay is between one and three hours.

***XTT Assay*** It was described by Scudiero et al. It uses the tetrazolium salt XTT (2,3-bis (2-methoxy-4-nitro-5-sulfophenyl)-5-carboxanilide-2H-tetrazolium, monosodium salt). While MTT produced a water-insoluble orange color formazan compound which required dissolving the dye in order to measure its absorbance, the XTT produces a water-soluble dye. The procedure of XTT is simply for measuring proliferation and is therefore an excellent solution for quantitating cells and determining their viability. XTT is used to assay cell proliferation as response to different growth factors. It is also used for assaying cytotoxicity [12].

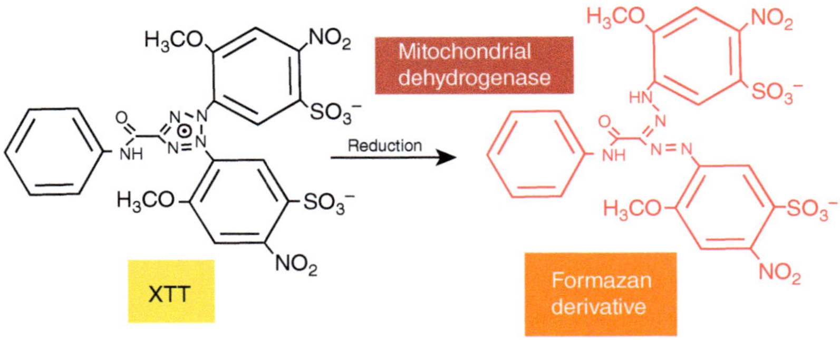


**Figure 4.5** XTT assay.

**Table 4.5** The advantages and disadvantages of in vitro, animal tests, and usage tests.

| Test | Advantages | Disadvantages |
|---|---|---|
| Initial tests | • Fast<br>• Inexpensive<br>• Easy standardization | • Limited simulation of a clinical scenario<br>• Lacks the ability to simulate complex interactions that exist in an organism |
| Animal tests | • Permits an intact biological system to respond to or interact with the tissues | • High cost<br>• Increased length of time<br>• Concerns regarding the ethical treatment of the test animals |
| Usage tests | • Clinical relevance is best achieved using these tests | • Complex study design<br>• High cost<br>• Long-term follow-up may result in patient fall out<br>• May involve legal and confidentiality issues |

**Advantages**: XTT assay can measure a large number of samples. No additional step for solubilization is needed. It has high sensitivity and accuracy.

**Disadvantages**: XTT assay performance depends on reductive capacity of viable cells with the mitochondrial dehydrogenase activity. Therefore, changes of reductive capacity of viable cells resulting from enzymatic regulation, pH, cellular ion concentration (e.g. sodium, calcium, potassium), cell cycle variation, or other environmental factors may affect the final absorbance reading (as shown in Figure 4.5).

***WST-1 Assay*** WST-1 (2-(4-iodophenyl)-3-(4-nitrophenyl)-5-(2,4-disulfophenyl)-2H tetrazolium monosodium salt) cell proliferation assay is based on the conversion of the tetrazolium salt WST-1 into a highly water-soluble formazan by mitochondrial dehydrogenase enzymes in the presence of intermediate electron acceptor, such as mPMS (1-methoxy-5-methyl-phenazinium methyl sulfate). The water-soluble salt is released into the cell culture medium [13].

To perform the assay, the WST-1 reagent is added directly into the media of cells cultured in multiwell plates. The cultures are then given 30 minutes to 5 hours to reduce the reagent into the dye form. The plate is then immediately read at 450 nm with a reference reading at 630 nm [13].

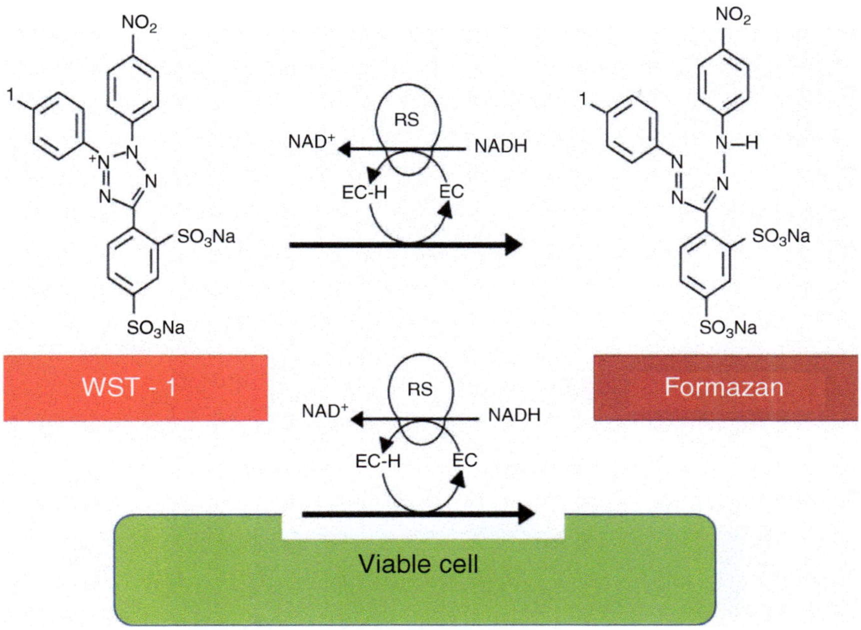


**Figure 4.6** WST 1 assay.

**Advantages**: It is easy to use, is safe and has a high reproducibility. As the colored dye produced at the end of experiment is water-soluble, it does not require a solvent and additional incubation time.

**Disadvantages**: The standard incubation time of WST-1 time is two hours. Whether one-time addition of WST-1 can reflect the effect of the testing agents at different time points on the trend of relative cell viability is still unclear (as shown in Figure 4.6).

***WST-8 Assay*** WST-8 (2-(2-methoxy-4-nitrophenyl)-3-(4-nitrophenyl)-5-(2,4-disulfophenyl)-2*H* tetrazolium, monosodium salt), a highly stable and water-soluble WST, is utilized in Cell Counting Kit-8 (CCK-8). It is more sensitive than WST-1 particularly at neutral pH. Because of the electron mediator, 1-methoxy PMS in this kit is highly stable, and CCK-8 is stable for at least six months at the room temperature and for one year at 0–5 °C (as shown in Figure 4.7) [13].

**Advantages**: WST-8 is not cell permeable, which results in low cytotoxicity. Therefore, after the assay, it is possible to continue further experiments using the same cells. Furthermore, it produces the water-soluble formazan upon cellular reduction, which would provide an additional advantage to the method by allowing a simpler assay procedure and not required an extra step to dissolve the formazan.

**Disadvantages**: An important consideration is that reduction of assay substrates is impacted by changes in intracellular metabolic activity that has no direct effect on overall cell viability.

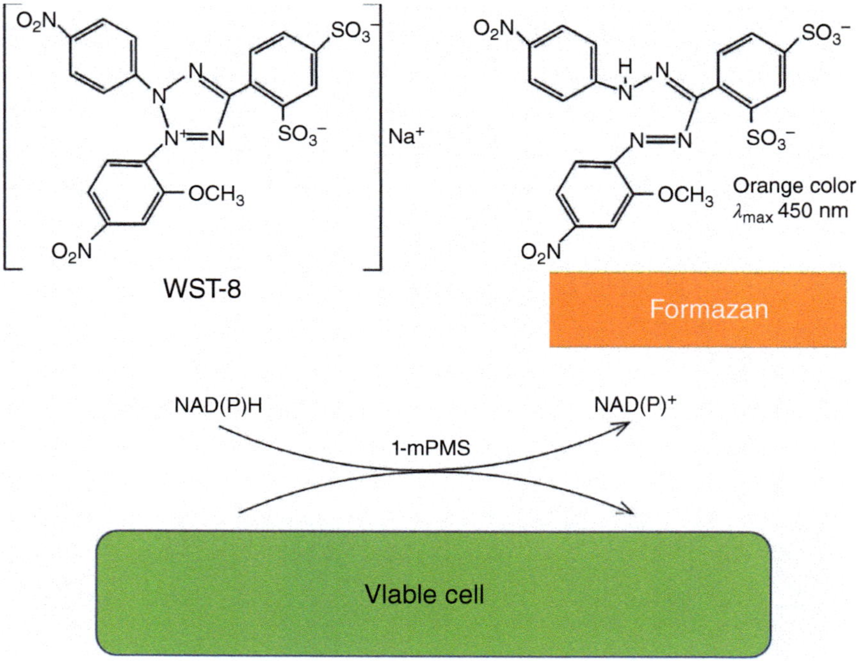


**Figure 4.7** WST 8 assay. *Source:* St John [13].

***LDH (Lactate Dehydrogenase) Assay*** LDH Cytotoxicity Assay measures the stable, cytosolic, LDH enzyme quantitatively. LDH is an enzyme that is normally found within the cell cytoplasm. With reduction in cell viability, leakiness of the plasma membrane increase and therefore LDH enzyme is released into the cell culture medium. The released LDH is measured with a coupled enzymatic reaction that results in the conversion of a tetrazolium salt (iodonitrotetrazolium (INT)) into a red color formazan by diaphorase [14].

The LDH activity is determined as NADH oxidation or INT reduction over a defined time period. The resulting red formazan absorbs maximally at 492 nm and can be measured quantitatively at 490 nm [14].

**Advantages**: This assay is an indicator of irreversible cell death due to cell membrane damage.

**Disadvantages**: The major limitation of this assay is that serum and some other compounds have inherent LDH activity. Therefore, this assay is limited to serum-free or low-serum conditions, limiting the assay culture period (depending on your cells' tolerance to low serum) and reducing the scope of the assay as it can no longer allow determination of cell death caused under normal growth conditions (as shown in Figure 4.8).

***SRB (Sulforhodamine B) Assay*** SRB assay was first described by Skehan in 1985. It was developed for use in the disease-orientated, large-scale anticancer drug discovery program of the National Cancer Institute (NCI). It is a rapid and sensitive colorimetric method for measuring the drug-induced cytotoxicity in both attached and suspension cell cultures.

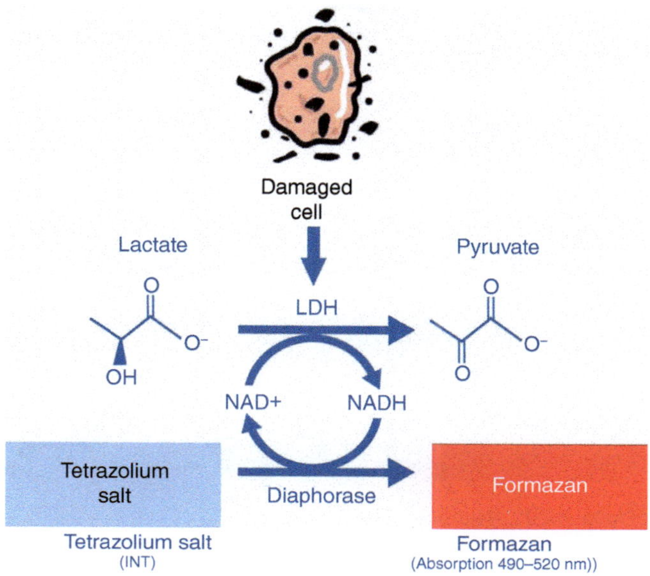


**Figure 4.8** Lactate dehydrogenase assay.

SRB is a bright pink aminoxanthene dye with two sulfonic groups. Under mildly acidic conditions, SRB binds to protein basic amino acid residues in trichloroacetic acid (TCA)-fixed cells to provide a sensitive index of cellular protein [14].

**Advantages**: The SRB assay is simple, fast and sensitive. It is less sensitive to environmental fluctuations and is independent of intermediary metabolism. Reproducibility of this assay is high.

**Disadvantages**: It is important to obtain and maintain a homogeneous cell suspension. Cellular clumps/aggregates should be avoided for high assay performance (as shown in Figure 4.9).

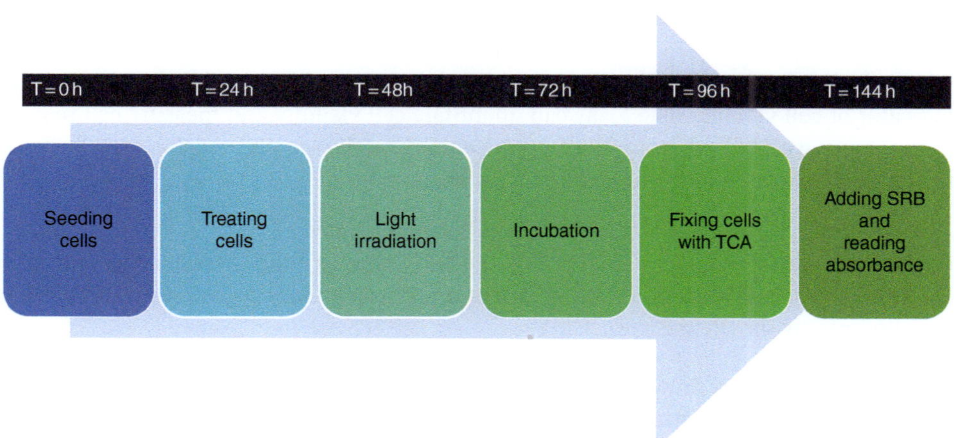


**Figure 4.9** SRB assay.

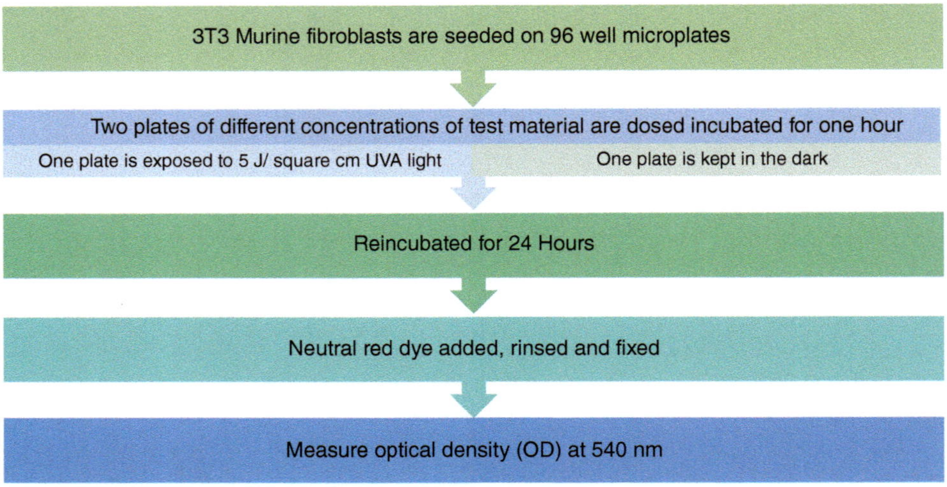


**Figure 4.10** Neutral red uptake assay.

***NRU (Neutral Red Uptake) Assay*** The NRU assay was developed by Borenfreund and Puerner. This assay is based on the ability of viable cells to take up the supravital dye neutral red. This weakly cationic dye penetrates cell membranes by nonionic passive diffusion and concentrates in the lysosomes. The dye is then extracted from the viable cells using an acidified ethanol solution, and the absorbance of the dye is measured using spectrophotometer [14].

NRU depends on the capacity of cells to maintain pH gradients through the ATP production. At physiological pH, net charge of the dye is zero. This charge enables the dye to penetrate the cell membranes. Inside the lysosomes, there is a proton gradient to maintain a pH lower than that of the cytoplasm. Thus, the dye becomes charged and is retained inside the lysosomes. When the cell dies or pH gradient is reduced, the dye cannot be retained. In addition, the uptake of neutral red by viable cells can be modified by alterations in cell surface or lysosomal membranes. Thus, it is possible to distinguish between viable, damaged, or dead cells. Lysosomal uptake of neutral red dye is a highly sensitive indicator of cell viability. The assay can quantitate cell viability and measure cell replication, cytostatic effects or cytotoxic effects depending on the seeding density. Absorbance is measured at 540 nm in multiwell plate reader spectrophotometer [14].

**Advantages**: NRR assay is a good marker of lysosomal damage.

**Disadvantages**: It has been reported that the NRR assay is either minimally or not at all affected by natural factors, such as temperature and salinity, but is mainly influenced by pollutants (as shown in Figure 4.10).

***CVS Assay (Crystal Violet Assay)*** In this assay, crystal violet dye binds to proteins and DNA of viable cells, and thus, attached cells are stained with this dye. Cells lose their adherence during cell death and are subsequently lost from the population of cells, reducing the amount of crystal violet staining in a culture [12, 13].

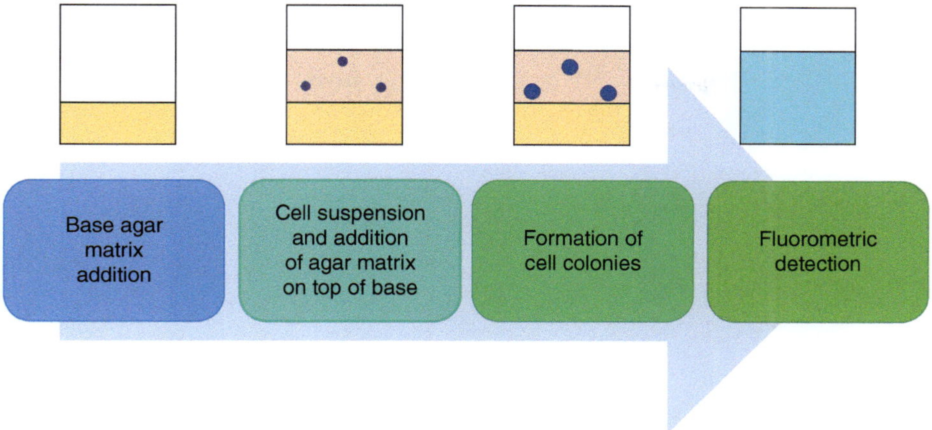


**Figure 4.11** Fluorometric assay. *Source:* Riss et al. [14] and Stanford [15].

**Advantages**: Crystal violet staining is a quick and versatile assay for screening cell viability under diverse stimulation such as chemical, organic, thermal, shock, and starvation of cells.

**Disadvantages**: CVS is insensitive to changes in cell metabolic activity. It is not able to measure cell proliferation rate as well.

#### 4.3.1.3 Fluorometric Assays

Fluorometric assays of cell viability and cytotoxicity are easy to perform with the use of a fluorescence microscope, fluorometer, fluorescence microplate reader, or flow cytometer. Fluorometric assays are also applicable for adherent or suspended cell lines and are easy to use. These assays are more sensitive than colorimetric assays (as shown in Figure 4.11) [14, 15].

***alamarBlue (AB) Assay*** AB assay is also known as resazurin reduction assay. The AB assay is based on the conversion of the blue nonfluorescent dye resazurin, which is converted to the pink fluorescent resorufin by mitochondrial and other enzymes such as diaphorases [15, 16].

Resazurin is a phenoxazin-3-one dye. Color of this compound is blue and it is nonfluorescent. After entering cells, resazurin is reduced to resorufin. Resorufin is red in color and highly fluorescent compound. Viable cells convert resazurin to resofurin continuously, increasing overall fluorescence and color of the cell culture medium. The quantity of produced resofurin is related to the number of viable cells. Ratio of viable cells can be quantified using a microplate reader fluorometer equipped with a 560-nm excitation/590-nm emission filter set. Resofurin can also be measured by absorbance changes. The incubation period required to generate a sufficient fluorescent signal above background is usually about one to four hours, depending on metabolic activity of the cells, the cell density per well and other conditions such as the culture medium type [16].

**Advantages**: AB (resazurin reduction) assay is relatively inexpensive and more sensitive than tetrazolium assays. Also, it can be combined with other methods such as measuring caspase activity to gather more information about the cytotoxicity mechanism.

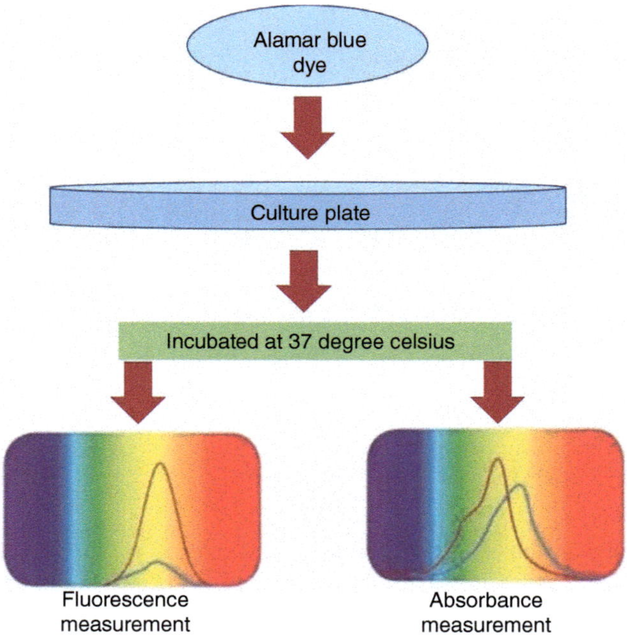


**Figure 4.12** alamarBlue assay.

**Disadvantages**: There maybe fluorescent interference from test compounds and direct toxic effects on the cells are possible (as shown in Figure 4.12).

***CFDA-AM Assay*** CFDA-AM (5-carboxyfluorescein diacetate, acetoxymethyl ester) is another fluorogenic dye that is an indicator for plasma membrane integrity. The dye CFDA-AM is a nontoxic esterase substrate that can be converted from a membrane permeable, nonpolar, nonfluorescent substance to polar, fluorescent dye, carboxyfluorescein (CF) by nonspecific esterases of viable cells. The conversion of CFDA-AM to CF by the cells indicate the integrity of plasma membrane, since only an intact membrane can maintain the cytoplasmic milieu which is needed to support esterase activity [17].

**Advantages**: CFDA-AM and AB assays were shown to be applicable on the same set of the cells, since both are nontoxic to cells, require similar incubation times and can be detected at different wavelengths without interferences.

**Disadvantages**: Fluorescent interference from test compounds is possible.

***Protease Viability Marker Assay (GF-AFC Assay)*** A cell-permeable fluorogenic protease substrate (glycylphenylalanyl-aminofluorocoumarin; GF-AFC) selectively detects protease activity which is restricted to viable cells. The GF-AFC substrate can penetrate viable cells. In these cells, cytoplasmic aminopeptidase activity removes the "gly" and "phe" amino acids to release aminofluorocoumarin (AFC) and produce a fluorescent signal proportional to the number of viable cells [18].

**Advantages**: It is relatively nontoxic to cells in culture. Also, at the end of the assay, cell population remains viable and can hence be used for subsequent assays. Furthermore,

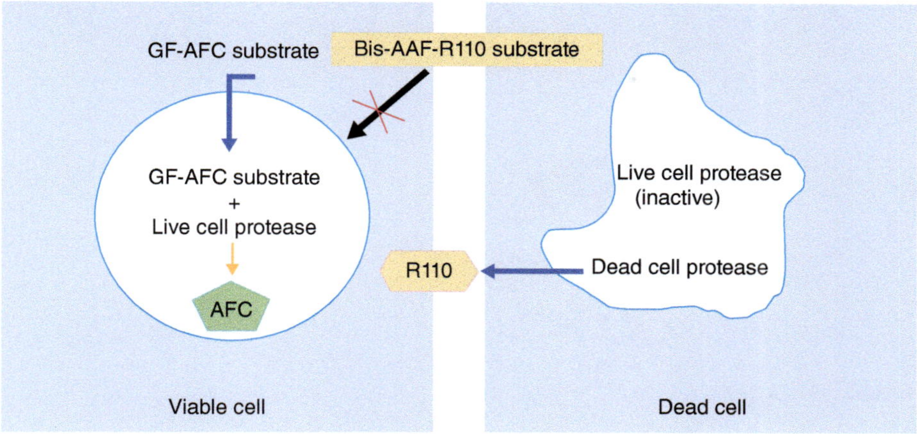


**Figure 4.13** Protease viability marker assay.

the incubation time is much shorter (30 minutes to 1 hour) compared to one to four hours required for the tetrazolium assays.

**Disadvantages**: Fluorescent interference from test compounds is possible (as shown in Figure 4.13).

#### 4.3.1.4 Luminometric Assays

Luminometric assays provide fast and simple determination of cell proliferation and cytotoxicity in mammalian cells. These assays can be performed in a convenient 96-well and 384-well microtiter plate format, and detection is carried out by luminometric microplate reader. A stable glow-type signal produced after reagent addition. This attribute can be harnessed to produce both viability and cytotoxicity values from the same well [19]. (as shown in Figure 4.14).

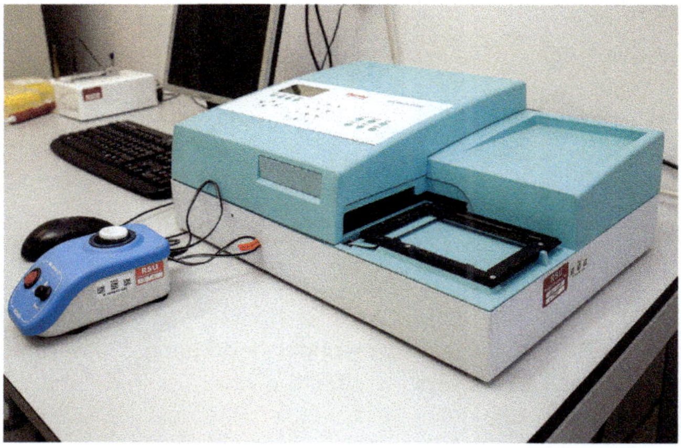

**Figure 4.14** Luminometric microplate reader.

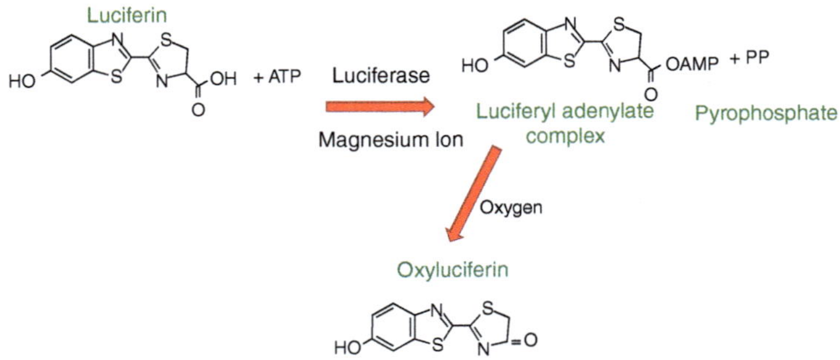


**Figure 4.15** ATP assay.

***ATP Assay*** ATP represents the chemical energy reservoir in cells. It takes part in biological synthesis, signaling, transport, and movement processes. Therefore, cellular ATP is one of the most sensitive end points in measuring cell viability. When cells are damaged lethally, they lose the ability to synthetize ATP and the ATP level of cells decreases dramatically. The ATP assay is based on the conversion of luciferin to oxyluciferin by the enzyme luciferase in the presence of $Mg^{2+}$ ions and ATP yielding a luminescent signal. There is a linear relationship between the intensity of luminescent signal and ATP concentration or cell number [20].

**Advantages**: ATP assay is the fastest cell viability assay to use, the most sensitive, and is less prone to artifacts than other viability assays.

**Disadvantages**: The ATP assay use limited as replicate samples need to pipetted which renders it technique sensitive (as shown in Figure 4.15).

***Real-Time Viability Assay*** In this assay, an engineered luciferase enzyme derived from a marine shrimp and a small molecule pro-substrate is used. The pro-substrate and luciferase are added directly to the cell culture medium as a reagent. Viable cells with an active metabolism reduce the pro-substrate into a substrate, which is used by luciferase, to generate a luminescent signal [21].

**Advantages**: This assay is the only assay which allows real-time measurement of cell viability.

**Disadvantages**: Eventual depletion of pro-substrate by metabolically active cells occurs with time.

**Things to Remember**

Luciferase is a generic term for the class of oxidative enzymes that produce bioluminescence, and is usually distinguished from a photoprotein. The name was first used by Raphaël Dubois who invented the words luciferin and luciferase, for the substrate and enzyme, respectively.

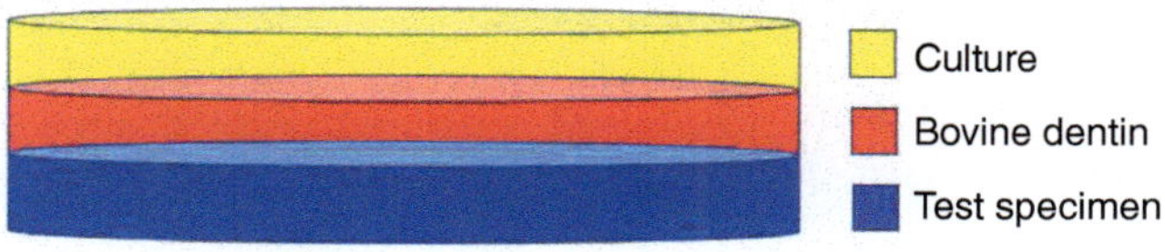


**Figure 4.16** Barrier screen test.

### 4.3.2 Barrier Screening Test

| **Good to Know** |
|---|
| Human and bovine enamel and dentine show the greatest similarity in terms of composition, structure, and properties. |

In this technique, a barrier of bovine dentin disc is positioned between the tested material and the cell culture. A positive cytotoxic response occurs if the material (or its by-products) penetrates the disc. This type of testing has a better simulation of the clinical scenario [22] (as shown in Figure 4.16).

### 4.3.3 Agar Diffusion Test

This test, also known as agar overlay or tissue culture overlay test, uses a layer of agar overlaid on a monoculture cell layer. The material to be tested is placed upon the agar layer. Dye used in this study is usually red vital stain. Identification of the toxic substance is evident as the presence of dye on the cell line indicates leaching [23] (as shown in Figure 4.17).

| **Things to Remember** |
|---|
| Agar diffusion technique is used for studying cytotoxicity imparted from the leachable components from the material. |

### 4.3.4 Filter Diffusion Testing Method

This method has close resemblance to the agar diffusion tests. A millipore (cellulose acetate) filter is interspersed between the primary cell line and tested material. Presence of any leachable component disseminates through a pore size of 0.45 µm to exert cytotoxic effects on the cell line [24].

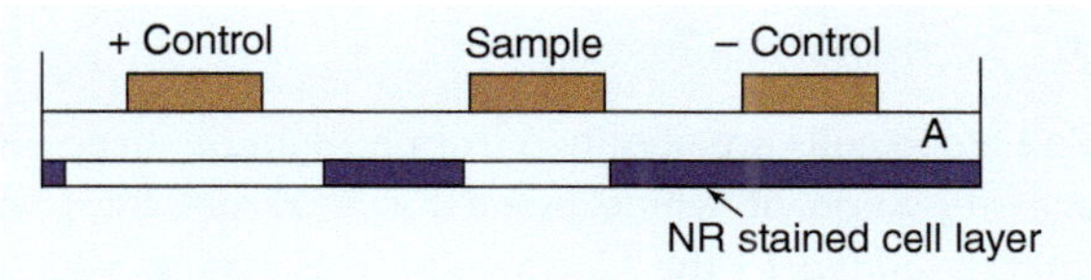


**Figure 4.17** Agar diffusion test. *Source:* Based on Guess et al. [23].

### 4.3.5 Tooth Slice Culture Assay

In this test, cultured slices of teeth that have retained pulp vitality are used. This test allows the role of cavity preparation and restoration variables to be measured.

| Good to Know |
|---|
| The tooth-on-a-chip is a novel platform that replicates near-physiologic conditions of the pulp–dentin interface and enables live cell imaging to study dental pulp cell response to biomaterials. The tooth-on-a-chip is made out of molded polydimethylsiloxane (PDMS) with a design consisting of two chambers separated by a dentin fragment. To characterize pulp cell responses to dental materials on-chip, stem cells from the apical papillas (SCAPs) were cultured in odontogenic medium and seeded onto the dentin surface, and observed using live cell microscopy. |

### 4.3.6 Micronuclei Test

The micronucleus is a small nucleus that forms whenever a chromosome or its fragment is not incorporated into one of the daughter nuclei during cell division. It is a test for genotoxicity. The experimental material is exposed to cell cultures of humans or rodents with and without an exogenous source of metabolic activation. The cells are then checked for micronuclei to assess the chromosome-damaging potential of a material [25].

### 4.3.7 Ame's Test

It was developed in the 1970 by Prof. Bruce Ames. Genetically altered strains of the bacteria *Salmonella tymphimurium* are used as test organisms which cannot grow on histidine-deficient agar medium. If the test material is mutagenic, then the bacteria will grow in the form of colonies on the surface, but if the test material is nonmutagenic, bacterial growth will not occur. The number of colonies indicates the degree of mutagenicity [26, 27] (as shown in Figure 4.18).

### 4.3.8 Style's Test

It is a modification of Ame's test that uses normal fibroblasts cultured from baby hamster kidney. Untransformed fibroblasts will not grow in an agar culture medium, whereas genetically transformed cells will grow beneath the agar medium [26].

### 4.3.9 Hemolysis Test

Red blood cells are obtained from human or sheep blood. Packed red cell is obtained after centrifugation of whole blood for 3000 rpm for 15 minutes. The sample to be tested is directly added to the blood cells in either powder or liquid form and then viability is assessed under the microscope.

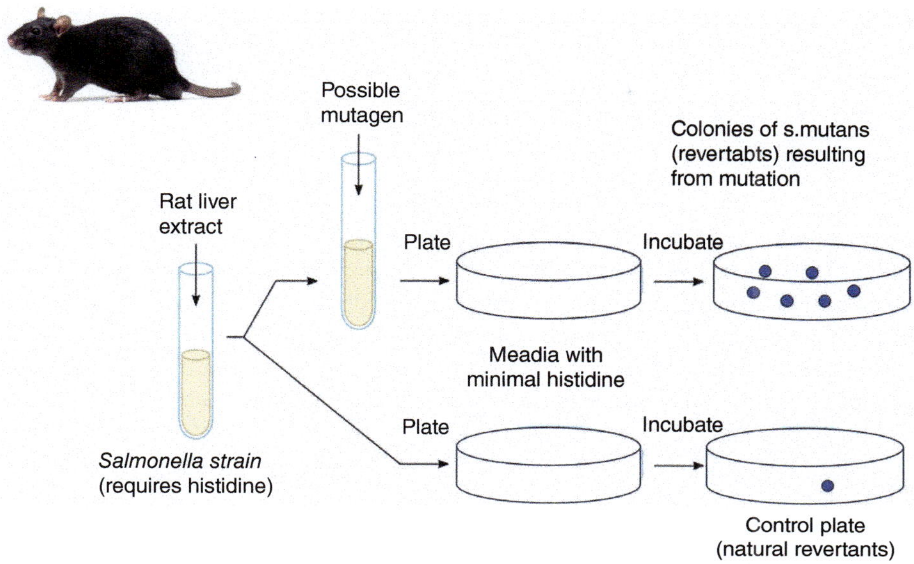


**Figure 4.18** Ame's test. *Source:* Tejs [26] and Maron and Ames [27].

## 4.4 Animal Tests

Animal testing is done to simulate a near-clinical scenario. Ferrets, dogs, monkeys, and rodents are the most commonly tested animals. The ISO 7405 guidelines classify the duration for testing as short term ($7 \pm 2$ days) and long term ($70 \pm 5$ days). Investigators prefer to split the duration between varied time intervals from 3 to 60 days or more. The cost can be a major limitation for adopting a short-time period. However, longer periods give a clue on the healing and regenerative responses [28].

The different types of tests are

i) Inhalation test
ii) Implantation test
iii) Maximization test
iv) Buehler's test

### 4.4.1 Inhalation Test

The tested material is sprayed near the mouth and chest of animals for 30 seconds. The testing continues thereon where for every half hour interval, the material is sprayed for 10 times. If the animal dies within three minutes, the material is considered extremely toxic. If not, a long-term follow-up is essential for the material to be described safe [29].

### 4.4.2 Implantation Test

The material is subcutaneously, intramuscularly or intraosseously implanted in the test specimen. Implantation periods can range from one week to many months. Following a short implantation test, about one to two weeks, inflammation adjoining the implanted material is evaluated. Intra-osseous implanted materials might use primates, dogs, pigs, guinea pigs, etc. Histological assessment of the tissue around the tested material is performed [29].

### 4.4.3 Maximization Test

For this test, a chemical called the Freund's Complete Adjuvant (FCA) is used. The primary form of this chemical is called the Freund's adjuvant. Addition of killed *Mycobacterium tuberculosis* to the primary form produces the FCA. The experimental material is intradermally injected into the animal with FCA and evaluated after seven days. On the seventh day, the same substance is topically applied for the next two days. After 14 days, the skin reactions are appraised. Care should be taken while performing this test, as the antigen, if applied in excessive quantities might lead to skin reactions and can be a confounding factor [30].

### 4.4.4 Buehler's Test

This test is very similar to the maximization test. The major advantage of this test is the elimination of the FCA component. The experimental animals suffer reduced damage due to the extirpation of the antigen [31].

## 4.5 Usage Tests

Usage tests can be performed in animals or humans. Animals that are large and have anatomical resemblance to human beings are used for this purpose. The test material is placed in an environment relevant to the use of the material in clinical practice. Clinical trials performed in humans are the highest rank of test for biocompatibility:

i) Pulp–dentin test for restorative materials;
ii) Pulp capping and pulpotomy material test;
iii) Mucosal damage and mucosa usage test;
iv) Periapical usage and endodontic damage test;
v) Gingival usage test;
vi) Teratogenic effects and influence on reproduction;
vii) Clinical trials.

### 4.5.1 Pulp–Dentin Test for Restorative Materials

This test is either conducted in experimental animals or on extracted human teeth. A class V cavity is prepared and restored. The material is kept under observation for weeks to months following which the pulp status is histologically evaluated [32].

### 4.5.2 Pulp Capping and Pulpotomy Material Test

It is a modification of the pulp–dentin test. Here, the material is placed directly on the exposed pulp to evaluate its role as a pulp capping and pulpotomy material [33, 34].

### 4.5.3 Mucosal Damage and Mucosa Usage Test

The inflammatory reactions to mucous membranes or abraded skin are tested. Hamsters are used for the test where the test material is placed in the cheek pouch and observed for any reactions after several weeks of contact. The pre- and postoperative photographs are compared, and biopsy specimens are analyzed for inflammatory changes [35].

### 4.5.4 Periapical Tissue Damage and Endodontic Usage Test

This test simulates a reaction that would be elicited following a conventional endodontic treatment. This animal model uses large animals such as primates or dogs. The evaluation is done by histological sections of the periapical region [36].

### 4.5.5 Gingival Usage Test

A subgingival cavity is prepared to ensure direct contact between the tested material and the gingiva. An evaluation period of around 7–30 days is required for this test [37].

### 4.5.6 Teratogenic Effects and Influence on Reproduction

These damages are to assess if a material can possibly elucidate any harmful effect on fetuses or newborns. The material is attached to the rodents prior to mating to both sexes or after mating to only females. The fetuses and newborns are evaluated microscopically and macroscopically for any aberration. This can be continued to the next generation as well to further survey any malformations [35].

### 4.5.7 Clinical Trials

A direct corroboration of the clinical performance and diagnostic tests on patients can be drawn by conducting clinical trials. It is imperative that the material clear the initial and the usage tests. Considerable legal and ethical considerations exist while performing these tests.

| Good to Know |
|---|
| The Clinical Trials Registry – India (CTRI) was launched in 2007 and is managed by the Indian Council of Medical Research (ICMR). The CTRI is an online, free searchable system for the prospective registration of all clinical trials being conducted in India. Registration of all regulatory clinical trials is mandatory as per the Drugs Controller General, India (DCGI). |

Once the material passes the in vitro and animal tests, the material is required to be approved by the Food and Drug Administration (FDA) of India prior to clinical trial.

There are four phases of clinical trial: [38]

1) **Phase I**: Material testing is done in a healthy individual. The increments are increased till an adverse reaction occurs. This determines the "Safety dose."
2) **Phase II**: Material testing is done in a small group of patients to determine the "therapeutic index."
3) **Phase III**: A large-scale study is conducted with control and test groups to prove the safety and effectiveness of the material.
4) **Phase IV**: Post-marketing surveillance.

#### 4.5.7.1 Clinical Testing of Restorative Materials

| Things to Remember |
|---|
| The Ryge criteria include assessment of marginal adaptation, anatomic form, surface roughness, secondary caries, and lustre of the restorative material. |

The clinical testing of restorative materials is evaluated according to the United States Public Health Service or Ryge criteria prior to commercial sales. The materials should be monitored for a prolonged period, i.e. one year, and also obtain a 90% success rate. In case of a deviation from either of the criteria, the test material should be withdrawn from sale. The scoring ranges from Alpha (perfect), Beta (not perfect, but clinically acceptable) and Charlie (restoration requires placement) to Delta (failure) [39].

#### 4.5.7.2 Allergy Tests

There are several types of allergy tests that can be performed on humans.

These tests are further divided as:

i) Patch test
ii) Prick test
iii) Radioallergosorbent test (RAST)

***Patch Test*** Jadassohn described the patch test.Allergens are loaded on to adhesive tapes at concentrations mildly high that would initiate a positive response and are attached to the patient's back. These reactions are mild, nonirritating, and essentially harmless. The classical signs include redness, itching, and blisters. Skin is evaluated followed by the removal of the patch after two to three days. A second evaluation after 7–10 days should be conducted to rule out delayed hypersensitivity responses. Patch test is to detect delayed hypersensitivity (Type IV) reactions. Skin and oral mucosa are comparable [40]. When the same test is performed at the actual site, in the oral cavity, it is termed as epidermal test. However, due to factors such as saliva and a mild discrepancy in the immunological reaction, the allergic response is not always elicited. A higher concentration may be necessary to overcome this problem [40] (as shown in Figure 4.19).

***Prick Test*** This test can be employed to detect an immediate-type allergic reaction or the Type I hypersensitivity reactions. The allergen is placed as a drop on the skin, and the skin

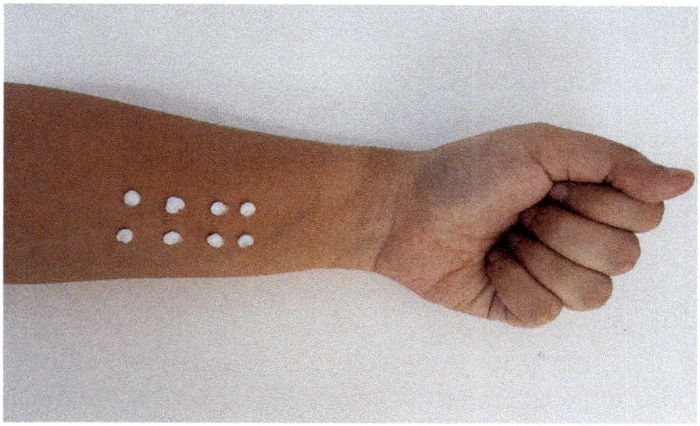

**Figure 4.19** Patch test.

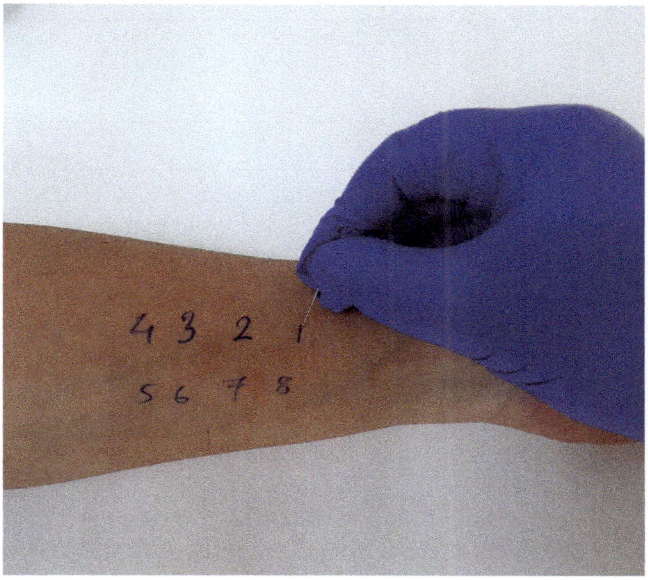


**Figure 4.20** Prick test.

is pierced through the drop. Presence of any positive reaction is detected after a period of 5–30 minutes [40]. In contrast to the patch test, the risk of sensitization is fairly low with prick test (as shown in Figure 4.20).

***Radioallergosorbent Test (RAST)*** This test was described in 1967 by Wide, Bennich, and Johansson. It is an in vitro substitute of prick test. It is used to detect immediate hypersensitivity. The allergen is linked to a material that is insoluble and the patient's serum is added. The allergen evokes a response by binding to the antibody if the added serum has antibodies to it. Radiolabelled IgE antibody is added to the allergen–serum mixture, and a complex reaction occurs with the already linked insoluble material. IgE antibodies that did not react and form a complex are washed away [41]. It is a quantitative test in the sense the linked radioactivity determines the amount of serum IgE released for a given allergen [41].

**Good to Know**

**According to FDA,** sample size varies based on the phase of testing prior to marketing.

**Early feasibility tests** are those which are carried out in the laboratory prior to human testing. They are used to form the initial safety data sheet of a material. **The sample size ranges from 10 to 15.**

**The pivotal study is done** to collect definitive evidence of the safety and effectiveness of a device for a specified intended use, typically in a **statistically justified number of subjects** prior to pre-marketing submission.

In India, if any material is to be tested for educational or exploratory purpose, then Institutional Ethical Committee (IEC) and ICMR are the regulatory bodies.

If a material is to be tested for commercial release, then Central Drugs Standard Control Organization (CDSCO) and ICMR are the regulatory bodies.

**Key Points**

1) Biocompatibility of dental materials is characterized by many parameters such as toxicity, allergenicity, genotoxicity, mutagenicity, carcinogenicity, and teratogenicity.
2) A series of in vitro and in vivo tests are conducted for the assessment of biocompatibility of a dental material.
3) The ANSI/ADA 41 and the ISO 10993 and ISO 7405 are the standards for the testing of biocompatibility of dental materials.
4) The biocompatibility tests are divided into three basic phases: primary phase (initial in vitro tests), secondary phase (animal tests) and usage phase (clinical scenario simulation).
5) Prior to animal and human testing, a material has to undergo a series of in vitro or laboratory test. Direct cell culture test, barrier screening test, agar diffusion testing, filter diffusion test, tooth slice culture assay, micronuclei test, Ame's test, Style's test, and hemolysis tests are the in vitro tests that are generally conducted.
6) Animal testing is done to simulate a near-clinical scenario. Ferrets, dogs, monkeys, and rodents are the most commonly tested animals. Inhalation test, implantation test, maximization test, and Buehler's test are done for animal testing.
7) Usage tests involve testing animals that are large and have anatomical resemblance to human beings. Clinical trials performed in humans are the highest rank of test for biocompatibility.
8) Amongst the allergy tests, patch test is used to test for delayed-type hypersensitivity reaction, Prick test is used for immediate hypersensitivity reaction and RAST is used for an in vitro test.

## References

1 Anusavice, K.J. (2004). *Phillips' Science of Dental Materials*, 11e. Sauders: Missouri.
2 Schmalz, G. and Bindslev, D.A. (2009). *Biocompatibility of Dental Materials*, 1e. Germany: Springer.
3 ISO 7405 (1996). Dentistry – Preclinical evaluation of biocompatibility of medical devices used in dentistry – Test methods for dental materials. International Standards Organization.
4 ISO 10993 (1992). Biological evaluation of dental devices. International Standards Organization.
5 Murray, P.E., García Godoy, C., and García Godoy, F. (2007). How is the biocompatibilty of dental biomaterials evaluated? *Med. Oral Patol. Oral Cir. Bucal.* 12: E258–E266.
6 Leirskar, J. and Helgeland, K. (1981). Mechanism of toxicity of dental materials. *Int. Endod. J.* 14: 42–47.
7 Kawahara, H., Shiota, M., and Yamakawa, Y. (1955). Studies on the effects of dental metals upon the mesenchymal cells in tissue culture. *J. Osaka Odontol. Soc.* 18: 343–348.
8 Schmalz, G. (1981). *Possibilities of a Standardized Test Using Cell Cultures*, 1e. Stuttart: Thieme.
9 Berridge, M.V. and Tan, A.S. (1993). Characterization of the cellular reduction of 3-(4,5-dimethylthiazol-2-yl)-2,5-diphenyltetrazolium bromide (MTT): subcellular localization, substrate dependence, and involvement of mitochondrial electron transport in MTT reduction. *Arch. Biochem. Biophys.* 303 (2): 474–482.
10 Cory, A., Owen, T., Barltrop, J., and Cory, J.G. (1991). Use of an aqueous soluble tetrazolium/formazan assay for cell growth assays in culture. *Cancer Commun.* 3 (7): 207–212.
11 Tominaga, H., Ishiyama, M., Ohseto, F. et al. (1999). A water-soluble tetrazolium salt useful for colorimetric cell viability assay. *Anal. Commun.* 36: 47–50.
12 Goodwin, C.J., Holt, S.J., Downes, S., and Marshall, N.J. (1995). Microculture tetrazolium assays: a comparison between two new tetrazolium salts, XTT and MTS. *J. Immunol. Methods* 179 (1): 95–103.
13 St John, K.R. (2007). Biocompatibility of dental materials. *Dent. Clin. North Am.* 51: 747–760, viii.
14 Riss, T., Niles, A., Moravec, R. et al. (2004). Cytotoxicity assays: in vitro methods to measure dead cells. 2019 May 1. In: *Assay Guidance Manual [Internet]* (eds. S. Markossian, G.S. Sittampalam, A. Grossman, et al.). Bethesda (MD): Eli Lilly & Company and the National Center for Advancing Translational Sciences.
15 Stanford, J.W. (1980). Recommended standard practices for cytotoxicity testing. *Dent. J.* 30: 141–173.
16 Rampersad, S.N. (2012). Multiple applications of Alamar Blue as an indicator of metabolic function and cellular health in cell viability bioassays. *Sensors (Basel)* 12 (9): 12347–12360. https://doi.org/10.3390/s120912347.
17 Bopp, S.K. and Lettieri, T. (2008). Comparison of four different colorimetric and fluorometric cytotoxicity assays in a zebrafish liver cell line. *BMC Pharmacol.* 8: 8.

**18** Niles, A.L., Moravec, R.A., Hesselberth, P.E. et al. (2007). A homogeneous assay to measure live and dead cells in the same sample by detecting different protease markers. *Anal. Biochem.* 366: 197–206.

**19** Aslantürk, Ö.S. (2017). in vitro cytotoxicity and cell viability assays: principles, advantages, and disadvantages, genotoxicity – a predictable risk to our actual world. *IntechOpen* https://doi.org/10.5772/intechopen.71923.

**20** Hall, M.P., Gruber, M.G., Hannah, R.R. et al. (1998). Stabilization of firefly luciferase using directed evolution. In: *Bioluminescence and Chemiluminescence—Perspectives for the 21st Century* (eds. A. Roda, M. Pazzagli, L.J. Kricka and P.E. Stanley), 392–395. Chichester, UK: John Wiley & Sons.

**21** Duellman, S.J., Zhou, W., Meisenheimer, P. et al. (2015). Bioluminescent, nonlytic, real-time cell viability assay and use in inhibitor screening. *Assay Drug Dev. Tech.* 13 (8): 456–465.

**22** Hensten-Pettersen, A. (1988). Comparison of the methods available for assessing cytotoxicity. *Int. Endod. J.* 21: 89–99.

**23** Guess, W.L., Rosenbluth, S.A., Schmidt, B., and Autian, J. (1965). Agar diffusion method for toxicity screening of plastics on cultured cell monolayers. *J. Pharm. Sci.* 54: 1545–1547.

**24** Kim, M.-j., Kim, K.-n., Lee, Y.-k., and Kim, K.-m. (2013). Cytotoxicity test of dentin bonding agents using millipore filters as dentin substitutes in a dentin barrier test. *Clin. Oral Invest.* 17 (6): 1489–1496.

**25** Sommer, S., Buraczewska, I., and Kruszewski, M. (2020). Micronucleus assay: the state of art, and future directions. *Int. J. Mol. Sci.* 21 (4): 1534.

**26** Tejs, S. (2008). The Ames test: a methodological short review. *Environ. Biotechnol.* 4: 1503.

**27** Maron, D.M. and Ames, B.N. (1983). Revised methods for the Salmonella mutagenicity test. *Mutat. Res.* 113: 173–215.

**28** Rowan, A. (1997). The benefits and ethics of animal research. *Sci. Am.* 276: 79. https://doi.org/10.1038/scientificamerican0297-79.

**29** Swetha, B., Mathew, S., Murthy, S. et al. (2015). Determination of biocompatibility: a review. *Int. Dent. Med. J. Adv. Res.* 1: 1–6.

**30** Sakaguchi, R.L. and Powers, J.M. (2012). *Craig's Restorative Dental Materials*, 13e. United States: Elsevier.

**31** Rowan, A.N. (1997). The benefits and ethics of animal research. *Sci. Am.* 276: 79.

**32** Smith, A.J., Tobias, R.S., Cassidy, N. et al. (1994). Odontoblast stimulation in ferrets by dentine matrix components. *Arch. Oral Biol.* 39: 13–22.

**33** Tziafas, D., Veis, A., and Alvanou, A. (1996). Inability of calcium hydroxide to induce reparative dentinogenesis at non-peripheral sites of dog dental pulp. *Eur. J. Oral Sci.* 104: 623–626.

**34** Kitasako, Y., Inokoshi, S., and Tagami, J. (1999). Effects of direct resin pulp capping techniques on short-term response of mechanically exposed pulps. *J. Dent.* 27: 257–263.

**35** Roy, M. and Wishe, H.I. (1986). Establishment of an improved implantation technique for hamster mucous membrane irritation testing. *J. Dent. Res.* 65 (11): 1365–1370.

**36** Kantarci, A., Hasturk, H., and Van Dyke, T.E. (2015). Animal models for periodontal regeneration and peri-implant responses. *Periodontology 2000* 68 (1): 66–82. https://doi.org/10.1111/prd.12052.

**37** Dablanca-Blanco, A.B., Blanco-Carrion, J., Martin-Biedma, B. et al. (2017). Management of large class II lesions in molars: how to restore and when to perform surgical crown lengthening? *Restor. Dent. Endod.* 42 (3): 240–252.

**38** Williams, D., Habib, A.G., and Warrell, D.A. (2018). Clinical studies of the effectiveness and safety of antivenoms. *Toxicon* 150: 1–10.

**39** Pardal, D. and Hegde, M. (2008). Clinical evaluation of different posterior composite restorative materials in class I and class II restorations: an in-vivo study. *Int. J. Dent. Sci.* 7: 1–8.

**40** Beltrani, V.S., Bernstein, I.L., Cohen, D.E., and Fonacier, L. (2006). Contact dermatitis: a practice parameter. *Ann. Aller. Asthma Immunol.* 97 (3 Suppl 2): S1–S38.

**41** Gleich, G.J. and Yunginger, J.W. (1981). The radioallergosorbent test: a method to measure IgE antibodies, IgG blocking antibodies, and the potency of allergy extracts. *Bull. N. Y. Acad. Med.* 57 (55): 9–67.

# 5

# Assessment of Optical Properties

| KEY CONCEPTS |
|---|
| • Knowledge of the three dimensions of color<br>• Dental clinic setting for color matching.<br>• Understanding of the importance and different methods of assessment of color stability.<br>• Insight into sample design for testing.<br>• Experimental setup for color stability assessment.<br>• Insight into fluorescence testing and gloss assessment. |

One of the quintessential challenges in restorative and esthetic dentistry is to produce a natural-looking restoration that blends harmoniously with the oral environment. Apart from the important parameters of shape and morphology, the color of a restoration is often regarded essential for constructing and maintaining as a "biomimetic" restoration.

Successful color matching in a restoration is one of the critical clinical requirements to increase acceptance of restorations. For a lasting impression of the esthetic outcome, color stability or the ability of the material to retain the matched shade with tooth over a long period of time is also crucial. Therefore, an understanding of color science and its parameters are important tools for optimizing the esthetic outcome of restoration. Furthermore, the science of color physics enables a quantification and comparison of color differences, which is an essential component in determining the color stability of material.

## 5.1 Perception of Color

"Color" is the quality of an object or substance with respect to light reflected by the object. In other words, color is the property of a surface or a substance due to the absorption of certain light rays and reflection of others within the range of wavelengths from 380 to 760 nm, which is adequate to excite the retinal receptors present in the eye [1].

Color perception depends upon the combination of three elements:

*Manual of Laboratory Testing Methods for Dental Restorative Materials*, First Edition.
Paromita Mazumdar and Deepshikha Chowdhury.

Companion website: www.wiley.com/go/mazumdar/dental-restorative-materials

1) Light source, which illuminates the object.
2) Object, which reflects, absorbs or transmits the incident light to the observer.
3) Observer, which perceives the reflected light.

## 5.2 Three Dimensions of Color

Color is usually described according to the Munsell color space [2] in terms of hue, value, and chroma. When color is to be determined using the Munsell system, value is determined first followed by chroma. Hue is determined last by matching with shade tabs of the value and chroma already determined (as shown in Figure 5.1).

### 5.2.1 Hue

Hue is the basic color. It is the quality that distinguishes one family of color from another. Hue is described with the words we normally think of as describing color: red, purple, blue, etc. It is specified as the dominant range of wavelengths in the visible spectrum that yields the perceived color, even though the exact wavelength of the perceived color may not be

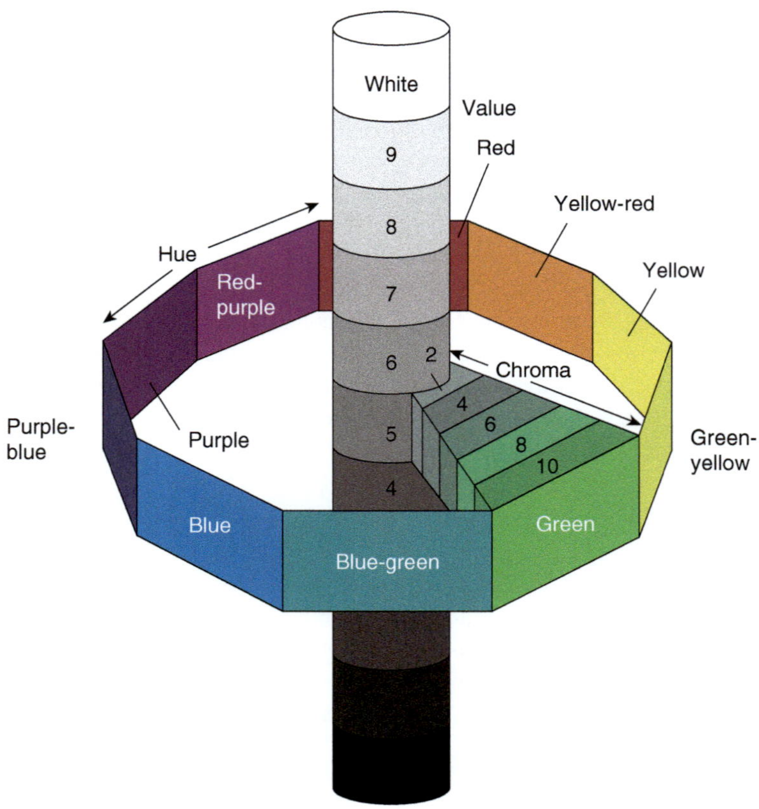


**Figure 5.1** Munsell color system.

present [3]. Hue is a physiologic and psychologic interpretation of a sum of wavelengths. Hue is represented by A, B, C, or D on the commonly used Vita Classic shade guide by student dentists and practicing dentists.

### 5.2.2 Value

"Value" is the lightness or brightness. It is the amount of light returned from an object. Munsell described value as a white to-black gray scale [3, 4]. Bright objects have lower amounts of gray and low-value objects have larger amounts of gray and will appear darker. The brightness of a crown is usually increased in two ways: by lowering chroma or by increasing the reflectivity of the surface. Lowering value means less light returns from the illuminated object and the remaining light is being absorbed or scattered elsewhere. While selecting colors, the correct lightness is selected followed by other color characteristics.

| **Things to Remember** |
|---|
| Value is the most critical of the three parameters when attempting to match an adjacent natural tooth; hue is the least important. |

### 5.2.3 Chroma

"Chroma" is the saturation, intensity, or strength of the Hue. If any dye (say red) is added into a glass of water and the same dye is added again and again, the intensity increases, but the color remains the same (hue). As more dye is added, the mixture appears darker; thus, the increase in chroma has a corresponding change in value. As chroma is increased, the value is decreased; chroma and value are inversely related [3, 4]. Higher numbers on the Vita Classic shade guide represent increased chroma.

To assess the value of the tooth, we look at whether the tooth appears light or dark. This perception is controlled by the amount of light reflected back to our eye after hitting the surface of the tooth. Value is intimately related to the surface morphology of the tooth. When light hits the surface of a tooth, the more the surface texture that is present, the greater the amount of the light reflected away from our eye. Therefore, the tooth appears darker or lower in value. In contrast, a smooth surface allows a larger amount of the light hitting the tooth surface to be reflected back to our eye and gives the tooth a lighter appearance, or higher value.

| **Things to Remember** |
|---|
| The VITA Classical A1-D4® shade guide (Vita North America, Yorba Linda, CA, USA) was introduced to dentistry in 1956. The VITA Classical A1-D4 is composed of 16 tabs. The tabs are arranged into four groups (A–D) based on hue with increasing chroma within the groups. In this arrangement, Group A is reddish-brown, Group B is reddish-yellow, |

*(Continued)*

**Things to Remember (Continued)**

Group C is gray, and Group D is reddish-gray. Chroma is categorized by numbers, i.e. 1 = least chromatic and 4 = most chromatic.

If we arrange the tabs based on value, they will be B1, A1, B2, D2, C1, C2, D4, A3, D3, A3.5, B4, C3, A4, and C4.

Vitapan 3D-Masterhas 11 sets of tabs, which consist of 26 sample ranging from lightest to darkest value, from lowest to highest intensity and from yellow to red. Samples are arranged in groups of 2 or 3 that form five sets (number 1–5). Each set shows a single value, 1 being the lightest (high value) and 5 being darkest (low value). In each of the groups, chroma increases from top to bottom (1 being least chromatic and 3 being most chromatic). All the group except 1 and 5 have 3 letters: L, M, and R, which allow hue to be chosen (L is yellow hue, M is yellow-red, and R is red hue) (as shown in Figures 5.2 and 5.3).

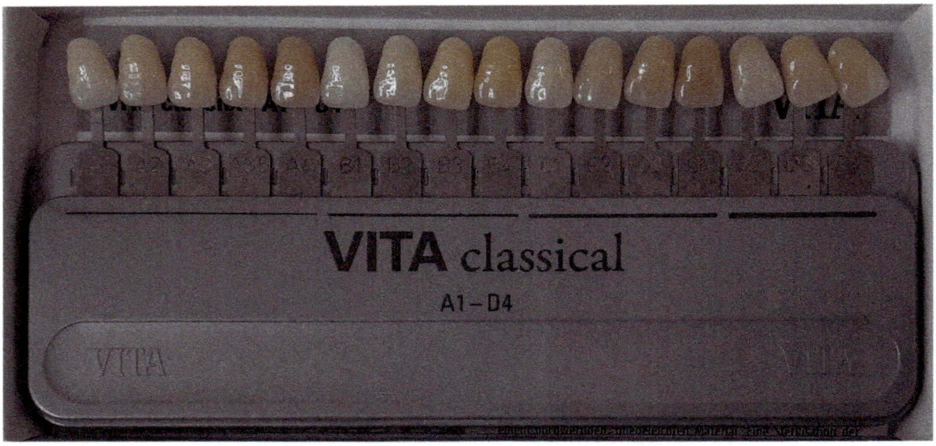


**Figure 5.2** Vita classical shade guide.

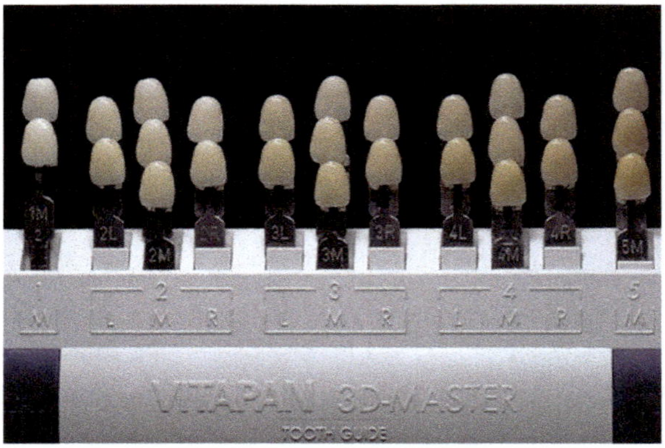


**Figure 5.3** Vita 3D master shade guide.

## 5.3 Color Measurements

Color measurements can be broadly classified into two categories – visual and instrumental color assessment [5, 6].

### 5.3.1 Visual Color Measurement

Subjective color identification usually involves a visual color assessment. It is commonly performed by visual comparison with reference color samples whose specification is known. In dentistry, shade guides are routinely used as the standard color samples against which a tooth or restoration is compared. Some of the popular shade guides are Vitapan Classical, Chromascope, and Vita System 3D Master. Visual measurements are generally easier to perform than instrumental measurements. However, one major criticism of these shade guides in the lack of a logical and ordered distribution in the natural tooth color space. A tooth contains more than 100 000 colors compared to the limited number of tabs in the shade guide, the probability of obtaining color match is approximately 1 in 100 000, assuming that the tooth and shade tabs contain only one color [7]. To have any realistic chance of obtaining a color match, the number of tabs in the shade guide would have to be increased to thousands, which is not possible practically.

| Good to Know |
|---|
| While shade selection, a black and white photograph of the selected shade in the patient's mouth gives a good clinical indication about value. |

### 5.3.2 Instrumental Color Measurement

This system, utilizes the Commission Internationale de l'Eclairage (CIE) system, where the color space consists of three coordinates: $L^*$, $a^*$, and $b^*$. The $L^*$ refers to the lightness coordinate, and its value ranges from 0 for perfect black to 100 for perfect white. The $a^*$ and $b^*$ are the chromaticity coordinates in the red–green axis and yellow–blue axis, respectively. Positive $a^*$ values reflect the red color range and negative values indicate the green color range. Similarly, positive $b^*$ values indicate the yellow color range, while negative values indicate the blue color range. The differences in the lightness and chromaticity coordinates ($\Delta L^*$, $\Delta a^*$, and $\Delta b^*$) as a result of ultraviolet (UV) light exposure are determined first, and the total color change ($\Delta E^*ab$) can be calculated using the relationship (as shown in Figure 5.4):

$$\Delta E = \left(\Delta l^2 + \Delta a^2 + \Delta b^2\right)^{1/2} \qquad (5.1)$$

Instrumental color analysis offers a potential advantage over visual color determination because instrumental readings are objective, can be quantified and are more rapidly obtained [8–10].

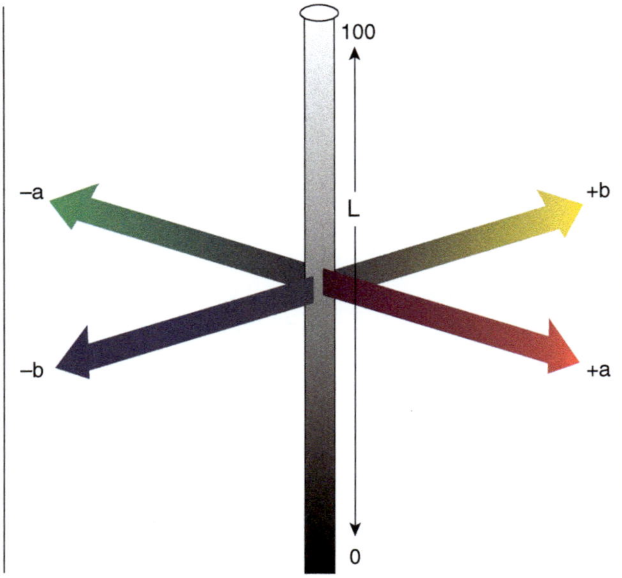


**Figure 5.4** CIE lab system.

There are three main categories of instruments used for color assessment:

1) Colorimeters,
2) Spectrophotometers
3) Digital imaging system

Spectrophotometers and colorimeters have been used with modifications in an attempt to overcome the problems with visual shade matching in dentistry.

**Colorimeter:** A colorimeter quantifies color by measuring three primary color components of light which corresponds to physiological trichromatic nature of the normal eye. It measures color with the help of a standard light source (illuminant), the subject, the detector and interpreter. The light created by the light source passes through the subject where some light is usually absorbed, is received by the sensor and is interpreted into an output such as a CIE chromacity graph. Photoelectric tristimulus colorimeters have the potential to remove some of the shortcomings of the visual method and have been shown to provide accurate and repeatable measurements; however, they are not entirely free of errors [11, 12].

**Spectrophotometer:** Spectrophotometers are instruments designed to produce the most accurate color measurements. There are two types of basic designs commonly used for these instruments. The traditional scanning instrument consists of a single photodiode detector that records the amount of light at each wavelength. The light is divided into small wavelength intervals by passing it through a monochromator. A more recent design uses a diode array with a dedicated element for each wavelength. This design allows for the simultaneous integration of all wavelengths. Both designs are considerably slower than filter colorimeters. Vita EasyShade is an example of a spectrophotometer [11, 12].

**Digital imaging system:** In dentistry, the instrumental color measurement also encompasses imaging system. With an appropriate calibration protocol (e.g. object–camera distance, digital camera settings, and suitable illumination coordinates), the digital imaging method has been suggested as an alternative color measurement tool with reasonable accuracy and reliability.

The help of mathematical calculation enables color to be identified by numbers, and color differences can be measured and thus quantified. These measurements also allow one to quantify and analyze which parameters of color (hue, value, and chroma) have changed and to what extent [13, 14].

Recent advances in photography and computing have resulted in the widespread use of the digital camera for color imaging. This new technique is capable of recording digital data from an object, which may subsequently be used to produce an image when viewed on a computer and which may be transmitted via the Internet. Images produced via a digital camera may be analyzed using appropriate imaging software enabling the collection of color values from the whole or parts of such images. This is a more convenient and economical process than the use of traditional color measurement devices such as spectrophotometers or colorimeters.

The color stability of a dental restoration is crucial for dental professionals and patients. In fact, the quality of a restoration is considered from both functional and esthetic points of view. The search for ideal esthetic and functional restoratives resulted in significant improvements in materials and techniques over time. Long-term exposure to staining media from food items can significantly affect the color stability of modern esthetic restorative materials regardless of different compositions. Hence, color stability is an important property which must be assessed.

Shade matching is one of the criteria for the assessment of restoration quality according to the "Modified Ryge Criteria." It is important because eventually the laboratory findings are to be related clinically [15].

**Good to Know**

The properties of translucence, fluorescence and opalescence are important in esthetic dentistry to replicate the enamel.

Translucence is the ability of the light to partially pass through an object.

Fluorescence is the ability to absorb light of a particular and is reemitted as a light of longer wavelength.

Opalescence is the ability of the object to appear blue or red in reflected or transmitted light.

## 5.4 Experimental Design for the Assessment of Color Stability

1) Sample preparation
2) Staining procedure
3) Assessment of color change

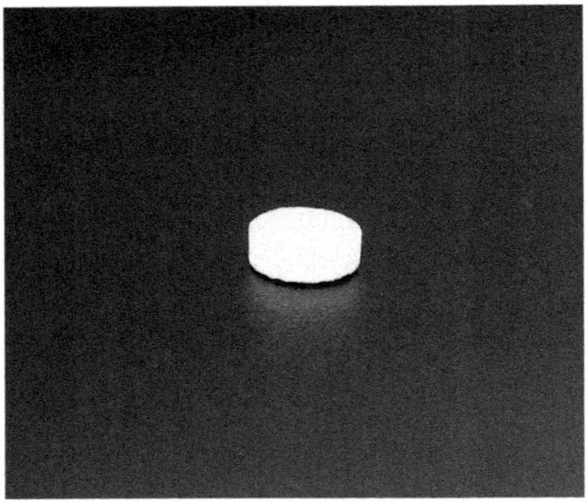

**Figure 5.5** Composite resin specimen.

### 5.4.1 Sample Preparation for Color Stability Assessment

| Good to Know |
|---|
| Since distilled water is non-ionized water, there is no chemical reaction with the restorative material thus preventing disturbance in the surface properties of the material. |

Disc-shaped specimens having a thickness of 2 mm and a minimum diameter of 5 mm and a maximum diameter of 25 mm must be fabricated (as shown in Figure 5.5). The material for the mold may be Teflon or silicon or polyethylene plastic that may be cut out from polyethylene pipes in order to facilitate easy placement of the unset or uncured material and removal of the set or cured material. The specimens are then immersed in distilled water at 37 °C for 24 hours in an incubator. For the constant maintenance of temperature in the incubator, a thermometer is used to check that the thermostat functioning efficiently.

### 5.4.2 Staining Procedure

Staining solution may be beverages such as tea, coffee, fruit juices, red wine, chocolates, turmeric, berries, or other colored substances that are consumed and having varying contact period with teeth, mucosal surfaces and tongue.

The specimens are then immersed in the staining solutions at 37°C over the test period to simulate oral conditions. The process of immersion may be for a continuous time period or may be periodic, thereby simulating clinic situations. Solutions must be changed daily and put in amber color glass vials with cover that prevent evaporation of staining solutions. The vials must be labeled in order to carry out experimentation efficiently.

### 5.4.3 Assessment of Color Change

1) **Visual assessment:** Shade matching is accomplished by visually comparing a tooth with multiple standards, usually represented as shade guide tabs. Factors such as observer color perception, observer bias, ambient lighting, and the acceptance

threshold of mismatch have effects on value, hue, and chroma present in human tooth structure.

2) **Colorimetric analysis:** A colorimeter is a device of fairly simple design based upon the visual concepts of color. The sample is illuminated at a 45° angle relative to the perpendicular line to the plane of the mounted sample. The reflected light is measured directly perpendicular to the sample through a series of three and sometimes four colored filters which represent the relative amounts of red, green, and blue light reflected from the sample. More specifically, these filters are designed to ideally simulate the three functions, $x$, $y$, and $z$, for the Standard Observer so that the instrument directly measures the three tristimulus values, $X$, $Y$, and $Z$, for the specific illuminant being used [14]. Filter colorimeters generally use three or four silicon photodiodes that have spectral correction filters. These filters act as analog function generators that limit the spectral characteristics of the light striking the detector surface. Because of their consistent and rapid sensing nature, these devices can be used for quality control. ShadeEye is an example of a colorimeter based on the natural color concept (as shown in Figure 5.6).
3) **Spectrophotometric analysis:** Spectrophotometers differ from colorimeters in that they measure reflectance, transmittance or absorbance for various wavelengths in the spectrum [13, 14]. In the case of reflectance measurement, the quantity measured is termed Reflectance Factor and is defined as the reflectance of the sample at a given wavelength compared to the reflectance of the perfect diffuse white measured under the exact same conditions.

Both colorimeters and spectrophotometers have ease of handling which enables the objectification of color coordinates in a matter of seconds thereby increasing the measurement accuracy (as shown in Figure 5.7).

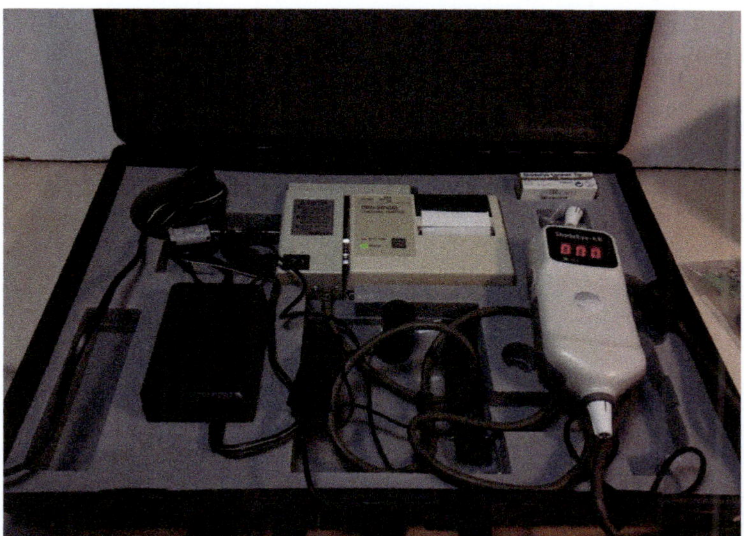

**Figure 5.6** ShadeEye colorimeter.

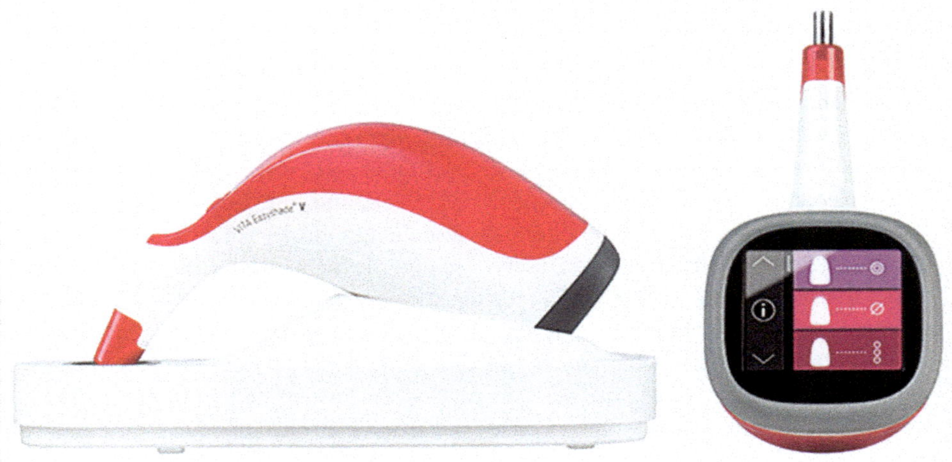

**Figure 5.7** Vita easy shade spectrophotometer.

4) **Digital image analysis**: The color stability of the specimens are assessed in the Commission International el' Eclairege $L^*a^*b^*$ (CIELAB) color space using a digital image analysis method. For digital color measurement, four light emitting diode (LED) bulbs (15 W each) are required to be mounted perpendicular to the frontal plane of the object having a distance of 15 cm from the specimen, reflecting at an angle of 45°. Specimens are placed over a neutral background. Digital images are obtained using a digital single-lens reflex camera (Nikon D5300, Nikon India Pvt. Ltd.) adjusted to auto white balance with a complementary metal oxide semiconductor (CMOS) sensor having 18.0 million effective pixels. Images are taken from the specimens in an object–lens distance of 10 cm in the macro mode using manual settings (aperture: f/11; shutter speed: 1/80 seconds). Digital images are then transferred to a personal computer (PC), and color values are calculated using a software program (Adobe Photoshop CS2, Adobe Systems Inc., CA, United States) [15].

   Image files are opened in Adobe Photoshop software. An area of specific diameter is selected from the middle third of the digital image of the specimen using the "circle marque" tool within the Adobe Photoshop software. An area is selected such that the position can be reproduced every time the measurement is made. The "histogram" window within the software is selected to obtain average color values of R, G, and B of the selected area (4 mm diameter). These R, G, and B values are converted to CIELAB color coordinates using Color Metric Converter software (Color Eng Inc., United States). The reason for using this conversion software is that in the Adobe Photoshop version used, it is found that $L^*$ values were given on a scale of 0–256 rather than 0–100 (as shown in Figure 5.8).

   For assessment of color in patients, there are devices that incorporate both colorimeter and digital imaging system such as Shade Vision X rite (as shown in Figure 5.9).

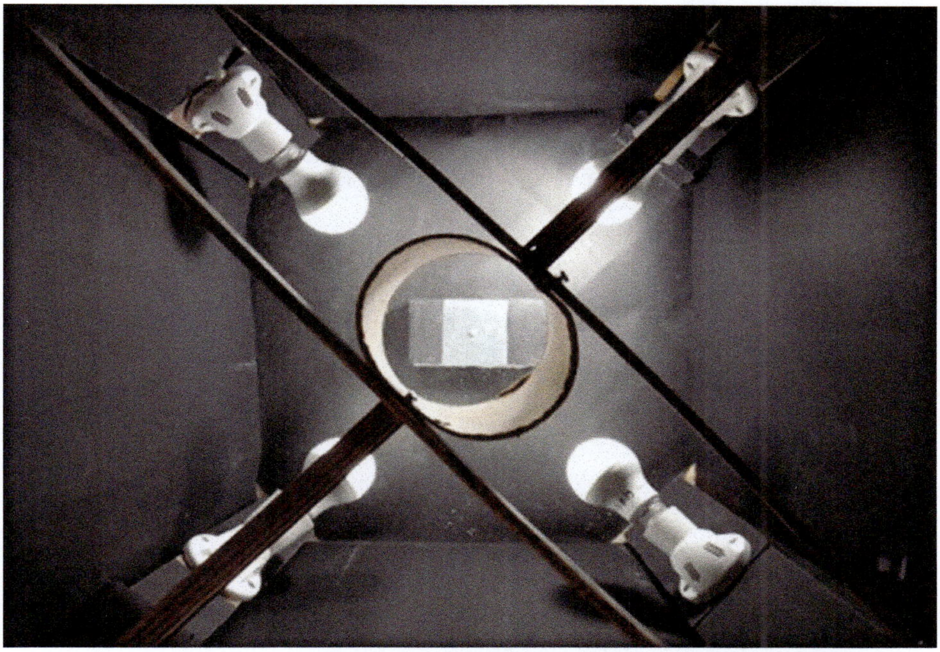

**Figure 5.8** Digital image analysis set up for laboratory assessment of color stability.

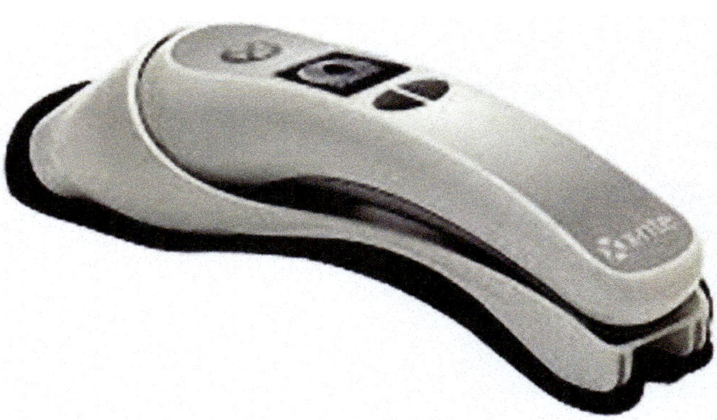

**Figure 5.9** X Rite colorimeter incorporated with digital imaging system.

## 5.5 Test for Color Stability of Composite Resin (Pictorial Representation)

For suitable performance, longevity, and good clinical success of esthetic restorations, the material of choice should present adequate inherent characteristics (Figures 5.10–5.16). However, the property of color stability of esthetic dental materials is often ignored over

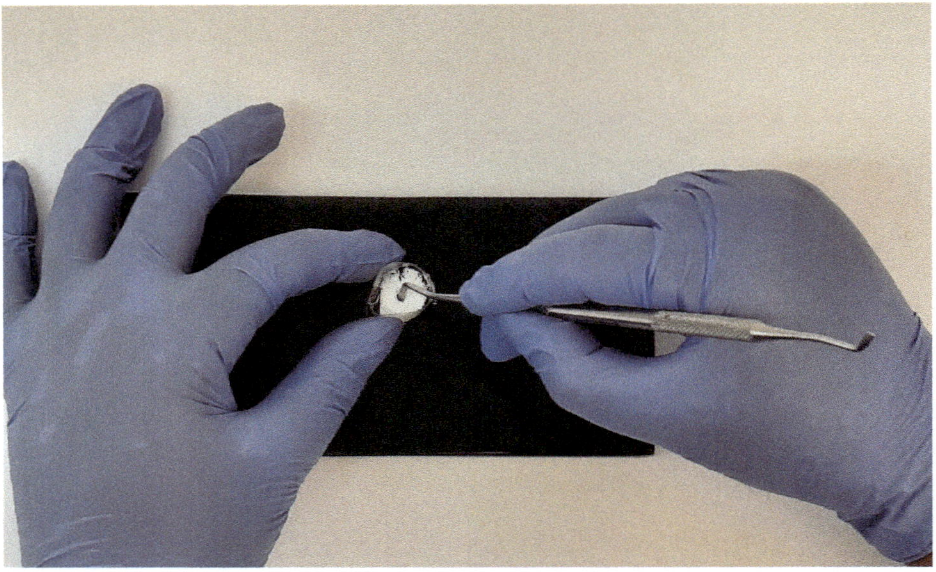

**Figure 5.10** Placement of composite resin in mold.

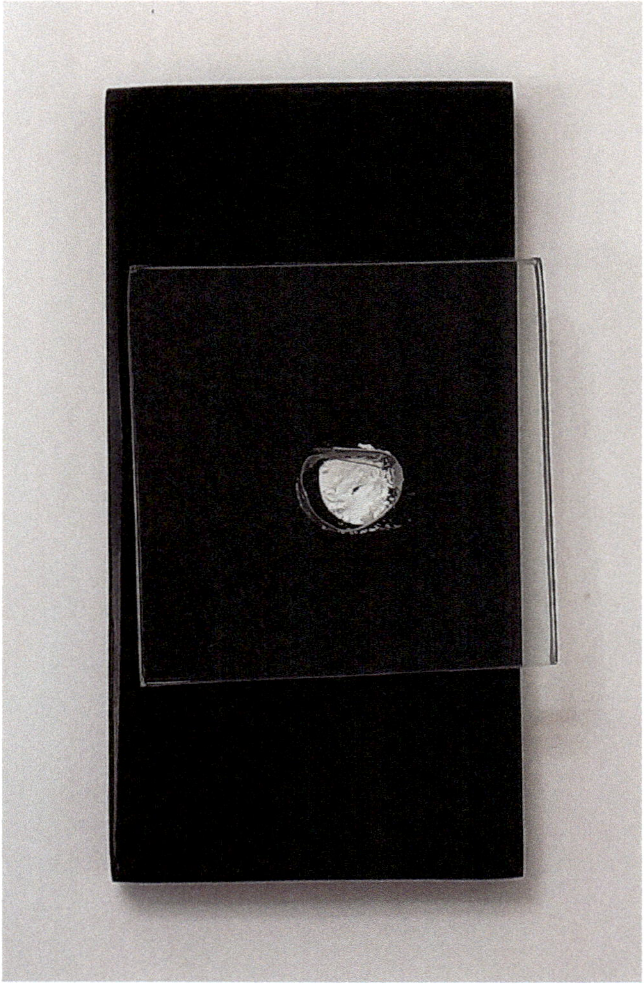

**Figure 5.11** Placement of glass slab over the uncured specimen.

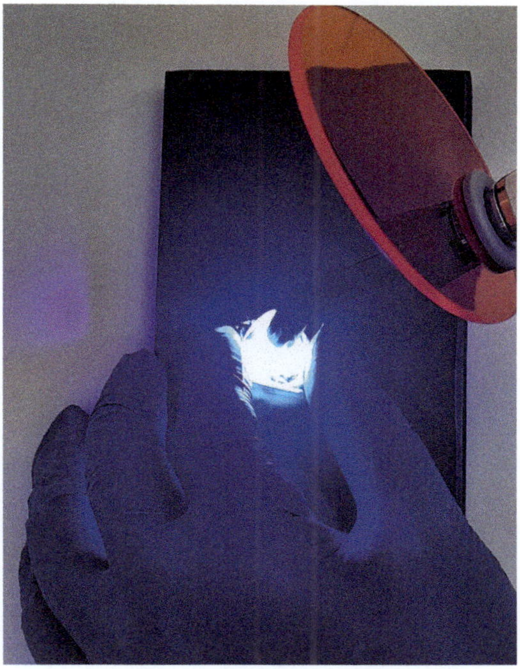

**Figure 5.12** Curing of the sample using LED light curing unit.

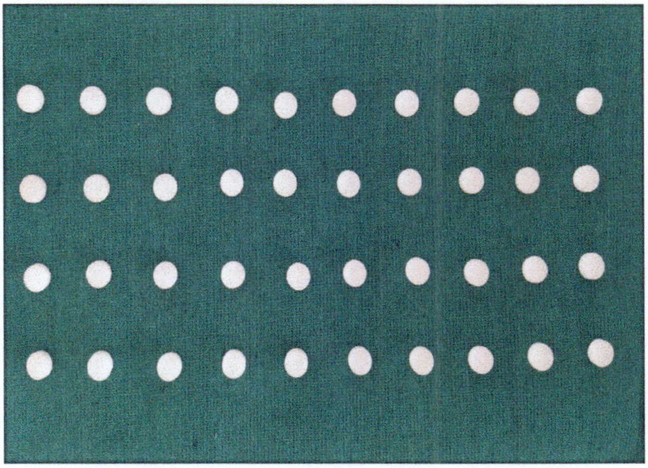

**Figure 5.13** Composite resin specimen.

other physical and mechanical properties while making a choice. The ideal esthetic restorative material formulations that may permit an optimal esthetic outcome without compromising the mechanical properties essential for a suitable functional outcome are nevertheless under exploration. It is imperative that an ideal restorative material should exhibit adequate esthetics as a function of color stability in addition to other properties such as strength and biocompatibility.

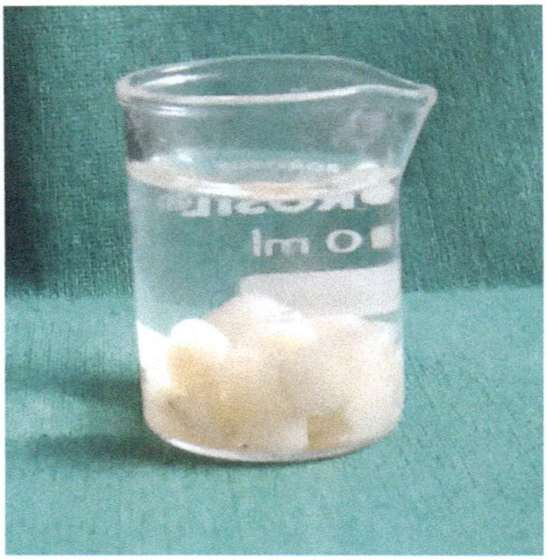

**Figure 5.14** Storage of specimens in distilled water.

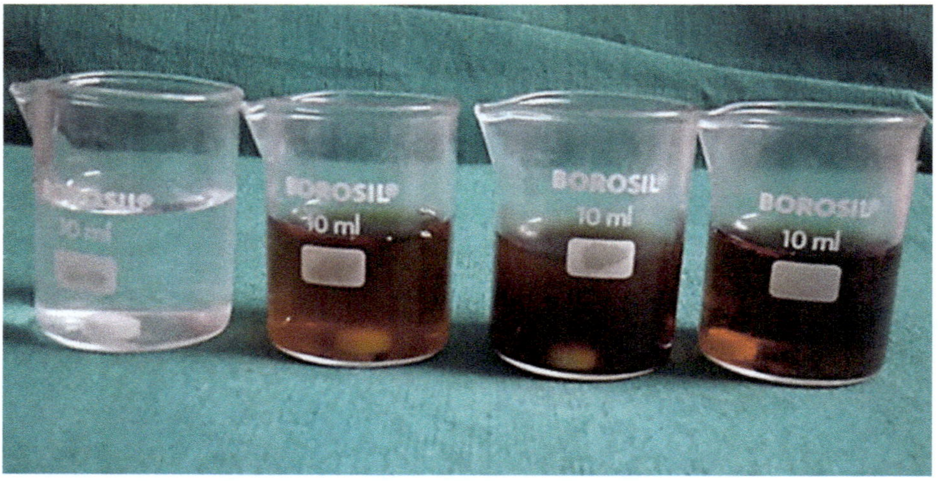


**Figure 5.15** Immersion in beverages.

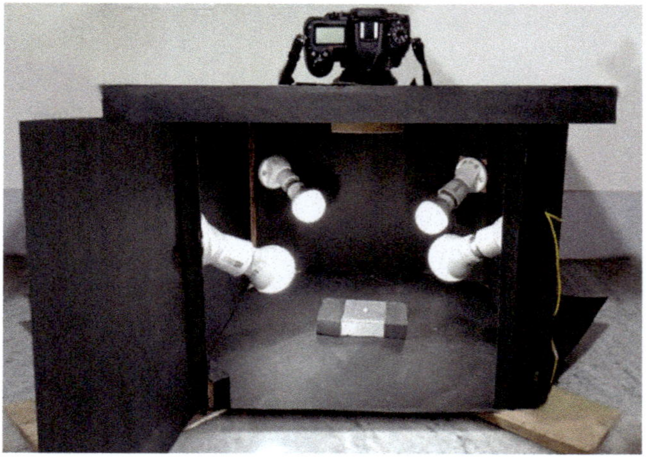

**Figure 5.16** Digital image analysis setup.

## 5.6 Assessment of Fluorescence

The role of tooth-colored restorative materials have substantially increased with patients having an increasing demand for esthetics. Apart from color stability, fluorescence is one of the optical properties of natural teeth that has attracted the attention of dental professionals in recent years. The reproduction of this property in esthetic restorations provides a visual perception much closer to reality, which makes these restorations more accepted by the patients. Shade matching allows the visualization of the restorative material under natural daylight, but it has to be taken into consideration that patients are exposed to varied light sources including large amount of UV light [16, 17].

Photoluminescence is the ability of a substance to emit light from electronically excited states immediately after the absorption of radiant energy. It is observed in all states of matter, both in organic and inorganic compounds. This phenomenon occurs through the absorption of photons followed by the spontaneous emission of new photons with less energy than those previously absorbed. Depending on the nature of the excited state, photoluminescence can be subdivided into phosphorescence and fluorescence [18].·

In phosphorescence, a transition from a triplet state to the ground state occurs and its emission rates are small, with long-lifetime emissions, which typically start milliseconds to seconds after the removal of the energy source [18, 19]·

In fluorescence, photon emission occurs from singlet states, and this allowed transition has emission rates much faster, with lifetimes near to 10 ns (10 × 10–9 seconds). A substance may exhibit phosphorescence, fluorescence or both, depending on the luminescent species in its composition [19].

The UV spectrum is divided into three regions: small, medium, and long waves. Long waves (UVA – 320–400 nm), popularly known as black light, are closer to the visible spectrum and are generally responsible for fluorescence phenomena [20, 21].

### 5.6.1 Fluorescnece of Natural Teeth

Human teeth are naturally fluorescent objects (also known as auto fluorescent) because UV light is easily absorbed by the luminescent species present in dental tissues. When UV light (between 350 and 400 nm) hits these tissues, it is initially absorbed and then emitted in the visible spectrum at longer wavelengths (between 410 and 500 nm). However, the amount of organic matter present in the tissue will dictate the fluorescence. Enamel produces weak fluorescence because it contains a small amount of organic material. Generally, teeth display a bluish-white color under UV light. The fluorescence spectrum of natural enamel exhibits maximum luminescence peaks at 450 nm, while the dentin shows peaks at 440 nm [22–25].

It has been seen that the fluorescence of dentin is mainly caused by the presence of a hydroxyapatite–pyridinoline complex. Several other organic compounds such as pyrimidine, tryptophan, tyrosine, hydroxypyridine, pyridinoline, and dityrosine are also responsible for fluorescence [26].

### 5.6.2 Fluorescence of Restorative Materials

Fluorescence contributes to the final appearance of esthetic restorations, by providing a closely mimicking clinical scenario in order to make the teeth and the restoration match as closely as possible. Since the basic components of dental resins and ceramics are not capable of promoting fluorescence, luminescent species have been added to improve this ability in the material. Inorganic rare-earth oxides such as europium oxides, cerium, terbium, ytterbium, dysprosium, and/or samarium are the most widely used agents. This improvement in fluorescence results from the mixing of several components at specific concentrations [27, 28]·

### 5.6.3 Measurement of Fluorescence

Fluorescence can be measured in several ways such as digital image analysis, fluorometers, and spectrophotometers.

**Digital image analysis:** The photographs are made under UV light using filters, so that the image obtained contains the information on the tooth and/or the tested material. They are digitally processed in an image software (e.g. Image J, MATLAB, or Origin) that analyzes the fluorescence image histogram of the restorative material and compares it with that of the adjacent dental area. When color photographs are analyzed, the fluorescence intensity (*I*) is calculated from the conversion of the color image to a grayscale [29].

The following equation has been used:

$$I¼0:299\,\mathrm{VR}+0:587\,\mathrm{VG}+0:114\,\mathrm{VB} \tag{5.2}$$

where VR, VG, and VB are the digital values of the red, green, and blue primary colors that make up the color of each pixel, where values lower than 0.06 are considered acceptable (the fluorescence of the material coincides with the fluorescence of the adjacent dental area) and values higher than 0.06 are not (the fluorescence of the material differs from the dental structure) [30–33].

**Fluorometers**: These are also known as spectrophotofluorometers, fluorospectrometers, or fluorescence spectrometers. These devices are used to measure fluorescence parameters, such as intensity and distribution, at various wavelengths. An emission spectrum corresponds to the wavelength intensity distribution of the emitted fluorescence, at a constant excitation wavelength. On the other hand, an excitation spectrum indicates the dependence of the emission intensity, measured on a single emission wavelength, when the excitation wavelength is varied [34, 35]. These spectra may be presented on different unit scales like energy (in eV) or wavenumber (in $\mathrm{cm}-1$), but the most usual is a wavelength scale (in nm). Fluorimeters have an excitation light source, most commonly a xenon lamp, which produces a continuous spectrum that starts in the UV region, covers all the visible region and extends to the near infrared. Two monochromators coupled to the equipment select the excitation and emission wavelengths, while the slits control the bandwidth of the light that passes the monochromators. The fluorescence is collected by light detectors, like photomultiplier tubes, charge-coupled devices (CCDs) or complementary metal-oxide-semiconductor, and is quantified by electronic devices. The results are displayed graphically and stored digitally. These devices can analyze liquid or solid samples. In the case of solid samples, the holder has a flexible metal rod that seizes the samples and, at the same time, allows them to be positioned in front-face geometry or, if right angle geometry is used, at 45° to the emission beam [36].

There are modern variations of these fluorometers where the fluorescence intensity can be obtained as a function of wavelength ($\lambda$), and three-dimensional (3D) spectra can be obtained from luminescence measurements based on excitation wavelengths in a 10-nm step. These multidimensional techniques provide a more comprehensive description of the fluorescence patterns because a total luminescence contour map is generated, functioning as a fingerprint for the identification and characterization of the material. In the 3D spectra, one axis represents the excitation wavelength, other the emission wave, and the third the fluorescence intensity. The acquisition of these maps requires numerous emission scans for each specimen. However, this analysis can be accelerated by CCD or video spectrofluorometers. The total fluorescence emission can be calculated as the volume below the fluorescence intensity surface, considering the emission and excitation planes [37–40].

**Spectrophotometers:** In general, a spectrometer is a device employed for acquiring optical spectra and can detect waves throughout the whole electromagnetic spectrum, from radio waves to gamma radiation. It measures and records the intensity of radiant light reflected from or transmitted from an object in a range of wavelengths. Its spectral bandwidth includes UV, visible and infra red (IR) ranges, and the most accurate models are those that have an integrating sphere, also known as spherical optics, in which the light reflected by the sample is collected at different angles and directions. The measured values for transmittance and reflectance are expressed as a percentage of the incident light power, while the absorbance is obtained from a simple mathematical operation over the transmittance. Its measurements can also be expressed in lightness ($L^*$), chromaticity a ($a^*$), and chromaticity b ($b^*$), which are the basis for calculating color differences in different colorimetric systems (e.g. CIEL*a*b* and CIEDE 2000) [41–43].

## 5.7 Assessment of Gloss

Esthetic restorative treatments strongly rely on the material's optical properties for accurate tooth mimicking. Besides the color of resin composites, it has also been reported that translucency, fluorescence, and surface gloss strongly affect the final result of esthetic restorations. Esthetic issues might be noticed when the resin gloss is different from dental enamel or other restoratives present in the mouth. Still, gloss is capable of altering color perception, which may favor restoration optical outcomes [44, 45].

Surface gloss is the optical property that produces a lustrous appearance [46]. There are several recognized gloss properties, including specular gloss, sheen, luster, and distinctness-of-image gloss [47].

In clinical practice, accurate restoration finishing and polishing might affect the way light reflects on the tooth surface, generating larger areas of reflection. This alters esthetics, especially the perception of tooth size and shape [48]. It is also known that restorations with increased roughness, besides causing esthetic problems, might also lead to greater biofilm retention [49–51]. Objective gloss (measured by a glossmeter) is the amount of light reflected on an object's surface at a determined angle and presenting the same angulation toward light incidence, but in the opposite direction, compared with a polished standard [52]. Although the objective gloss information is of extreme relevance to perform in vitro; studies, in clinical practice, objective gloss eligibility is unfeasible, given that teeth and/or restorations do not possess a perfectly flat surface (an important attribute for objective gloss interpretation). Furthermore, the subjective qualification of this property is routine in the dental field [53].

If surface gloss perception is targeted which is equivalent to the subjective gloss assessment, various aspects should be considered [54]. The visualization field, type of illuminant, surface characteristics of materials, color, and color of background may affect the perception of gloss. Usually for dental material gloss testing, the 60° measurement mode [55] is selected and the glossmeter is calibrated. Each specimen has to be centrally placed over the reading aperture of the machine. The light beam is transmitted to the surface of the material to be tested and reflected to the sensor. The measured area is square shaped (2×2 mm). After the first reading, the specimen in rotated 180° and a second reading is taken.

**Good to Know**

The steps for shade selection are

- Remove bright color from the working field. If the patient is wearing bright clothing, it is prudent to cover the patient with neutral color drape (grey). Any dark color lipstick should be removed because it could affect shade matching.
- Always clean the tooth using prophylaxis paste prior to shade selection.
- It is important not to view the shade comparison for more than 5–7 seconds to avoid eye fatigue.
- Clinician should be at a distance of 28–33 cm from the patient during shade selection.
- Always determine shade when the teeth are most hydrated because enamel dehydration reduces its translucency by 82%, misleading the clinician.
- Shade comparison should always be done in between 10 a.m. and 2 p.m. because at this time color temperature is around 5500 K. The commonly available source are natural daylight, incandescent light and fluorescent light. LED lights are also being used currently. Example of commercially available color-corrected lights are Demetron shade light and Vita-Lite.
- During the shade comparison, always place shade tabs either above or below the tooth to be match, never place shade tab adjacent to the tooth to avoid binocular effect.
- Always during shade selection, teeth should be divided into three regions: gingival area (gives accurate determination of dentinal chroma), body area and incisal area (enamel is thickest here and varies from translucent to transparent).

**Key Points**

1) Color is the quality of an object or substance with respect to light reflected by the object.
2) Color perception depends on the combination of three elements: light source, object, and observer.

3) Color is usually described according to the Munsell color space in terms of hue, value, and chroma.
4) **Hue** distinguishes one color from another and is described using common color names such as green, blue, red, yellow, etc. **Value** refers to the lightness or darkness of a color. It **defines** a color in terms of how close it is to white or black. **Chroma** is the attribute that expresses the saturation or intensity of a **color**.
5) Color measurements can be broadly classified into two categories: visual and instrumental color assessment.
6) Visual color measurement comprises of shade matching using shade guides.
7) Instrumental color measurement encompasses colorimeters, spectrophotometers and digital imaging technique.

## References


1 Brainard David, H., Cottaris Nicolas, P., and Ana, R. (2018). The perception of colour and material in naturalistic tasks. *Interface Focus* 8: 20180012–20180012.
2 Kuehni, R.G. (2002). The early development of the Munsell system. *Color. Res. Appl.* 27: 20–27.
3 Brewer, J.D., Wee, A., and Seghi, R. (2004). Advances in color matching. *Dent. Clin. N. Am.* 48: 341–358.
4 Stephen, J. (2002). Precision shade technology: contemporary strategies in shade selection. *Pract. Proced. Aesthet. Dent.* 14: 79–83.
5 Joiner, A. (2004). Tooth color: a review of the literature. *J. Dent.* 32: 3–12.
6 Paravina, R.D. (2002). Evaluation of newly developed visual shade matching apparatus. *Int. J. Prosthodont.* 15: 528–534.
7 Degarmo, E.P., Black, J., and Kohser, R.A. (2003). *Materials and Processes in Manufacturing*, 9e, 223. Wiley.
8 Sproull, R.C. (1973). Colour matching in dentistry II. Practical applications of the organization of colour. *J. Prosthet. Dent.* 29: 555–566.
9 Hall, N.R. (1991). Tooth colour selection: the application of colour science to dental colour matching. *Aust. Prosthodont. J.* 5: 41–46.
10 Johnston, W.M. (2009). Colour measurement in dentistry. *J. Dent.* 37: e2–e6.
11 Elter, A., Caniklioglu, B., Deger, S., and Ozen, J. (2005). The reliability of digital cameras for colour selection. *Int. J. Prosthodont.* 23 (5): 149–151.
12 Jarad, F.D., Albadn, S.S., and Mair, L.H. (2008). The use of objective digital matching to achieve an esthetic composite restoration. *J. Clin. Dent.* 19: 9–13.
13 Lath, D.L., Wilgoose, D.G., Guan, Y.H. et al. (2007). A digital image analysis for the assessment of tooth whiteness compared to visual shade matching. *J Clin Dent* 18: 17–20.
14 Caglar, A., Yamanel, K., Gulsahi, K. et al. (2010). Could digital imaging be an alternative for digital colourimeters? *Clin. Oral Investig.* 14: 713–718.
15 Guan, Y.H., Lath, D., Lilley, T.H. et al. (2005). The measurement of tooth whiteness by image analysis and spectrophotometry: a comparison. *J. Oral Rehabil.* 32: 7–15.

**16** Lakowicz, R. (2006). *Principles of Fluorescence Spectroscopy*, 3e. New York: Springer.

**17** Perrin, F. (1929). La fluorescence des solutions. Induction moléculaire— Polarisation et durée d'emission. Photochim. *Ann. Phys.* 10: 169–275.

**18** Svobodova, A., Walterova, D., and Vostalova, J. (2006). Ultraviolet light induced alteration to the skin. *Biomed. Pap. Med. Fac. Univ. Palacky Olomouc Czech Repub.* 150: 25–38.

**19** Abuduwali, N., Lossdörfer, S., Winter, J. et al. (2013). Autofluorescent characteristics of human periodontal ligament cells in vitro;. *Ann. Anat.* 195: 449–454.

**20** Foreman, P.C. (1980). The excitation and emission spectra of fluorescent components of human dentine. *Arch. Oral Biol.* 25: 641–647.

**21** Hoerman, K.C. and Mancewicz, S.A. (1964). Phosphorescence of calcified tissues. *Arch. Oral Biol.* 9: 517–534.

**22** Matsumoto, H., Kitamura, S., and Araki, T. (1999). Autofluorescence in human dentine in relation to age, tooth type and temperature measured by nanosecond time-resolved fluorescence microscopy. *Arch. Oral Biol.* 44: 309–318.

**23** Hall, J.B., Hefferren, J.J., and Olsen, N.H. (1970). Study of fluorescent characteristics of extracted human teeth by use of a clinical fluorometer. *J. Dent. Res.* 49: 1431–1436.

**24** Kvaal, S.I. and Solheim, T. (1995). Incremental lines in human dental cementum in relation to age. *Eur. J. Oral Sci.* 103: 225–230.

**25** Hafström-Björkman, U., Sundström, F., and ten Bosch, J.J. (1991). Fluorescence in dissolved fractions of human enamel. *Acta Odontol. Scand.* 49: 133–138.

**26** Da Silva, R.D., da Silva, M.A., de Oliveira, O.B. et al. (2013). Dental fluorescence: potential forensic use. *Forensic Sci. Int.* 231: 167–171.

**27** Takahashi, M.K., Vieira, S., Rached, R.N. et al. (2008). Fluorescence intensity of resin composites and dental tissues before and after accelerated aging: a comparative study. *Oper. Dent.* 33 (2): 189–195.

**28** Paula, S.S., Soares, L.E., Do Espírito Santo, A.M. et al. (2010). FT-Raman and energy dispersive X-ray fluorescence spectrometric analyses of enamel submitted to 38% hydrogen peroxide bleaching, an acidic beverage, and simulated brushing. *Photomed. Laser Surg.* 28: 391–396.

**29** Lee, Y.K. (2015). Fluorescence properties of human teeth and dental calculus for clinical applications. *J. Biomed. Opt.* 20: 040901.

**30** Tani, K., Watari, F., Uo, M., and Morita, M. (2003). Discrimination between composite resin and teeth using fluorescence properties. *Dent. Mater. J.* 22: 199–206.

**31** Rudd, K.D., Morrow, R.M., Welker, W.A., and Jendresen, M.D. (1967). Some uses of fluorescence in prosthodontics. *J. Prosthet. Dent.* 18: 543–549.

**32** Ecker, G.A., Moser, J.B., Wozniak, W.T., and Brinsden, G.I. (1985). Effect of repeated firing on fluorescence of porcelain-fused-to-metal porcelains. *J. Prosthet. Dent.* 54: 207–214.

**33** Baran, G.R., O'Brien, W.J., and Tien, T.Y. (1977). Colored emission of rare earth ions in a potassium feldspar glass. *J. Dent. Res.* 56: 1323–1329.

**34** Wozniak, W.T. and Moore, B.K. (1978). Luminescence spectra of dental porcelains. *J. Dent. Res.* 57: 971–974.

**35** Panzeri, H., Fernandes, L.T., and Minelli, A.J. (1977). Spectral fluorescence of direct anterior restorative materials. *Aust. Dent. J.* 22: 458–461.

**36** Reis, R.S.A., Casemiro, L.A., Carlino, G.V. et al. (2007). Evaluation of fluorescence of dental composites using contrast ratios to adjacent tooth structure. *J. Esthet. Restor. Dent.* 19: 199–207.

**37** Alves, L.P., Pilla, V., Murgo, D.O.A., and Munin, E. (2010). Core-shell quantum dots tailor the fluorescence of dental resin composites. *J. Dent.* 38: 149–152.

**38** Lefever, D., Mayoral, J.R., Mercade, M. et al. (2010). Optical integration and fluorescence: a comparison among restorative materials with spectrophotometric analysis. *Quintessence Int.* 41: 837–844.

**39** Torres, C.R., Ribeiro, C.F., Bresciani, E., and Borges, A.B. (2012). Influence of hydrogen peroxide bleaching gels on color, opacity, and fluorescence of composite resins. *Oper. Dent.* 37 (5): 526–531.

**40** Meller, C. and Klein, C. (2012). Fluorescence properties of commercial composite resin restorative materials in dentistry. *Dent. Mater. J.* 31: 916–923.

**41** Bueno, R.P., Salomone, P., Villetti, M.A., and Pozzobon, R.T. (2013). Effect of bleaching agents on the fluorescence of composite resins. *Eur. J. Esthet. Dent.* 8: 582–591.

**42** Lefever, D., Perakis, N., Roig, M. et al. (2012). The effect of toothbrushing on surface gloss of resin composites. *Am. J. Dent.* 25 (1): 54–58.

**43** de Alencar, E., Silva Leite, M.L., da Cunha Medeiros, E. et al. (2014). The effect of drinks on color stability and surface roughness of nanocomposites. *Eur. J. Dent.* 8 (3): 330–336.

**44** Başeren, M. (2004). Surface roughness of nanofill and nanohybrid composite resin and ormocer-based tooth-colored restorative materials after several finishing and polishing procedures. *J. Biomater. Appl.* 19: 121–134.

**45** O'Brien, W.J., Johnston, W.M., Fanian, F., and Lambert, L. (1984). The surface roughness and gloss of composites. *J. Dent. Res.* 63 (5): 685–688.

**46** Hunter, R.S. (1975). *The Measurement of Appearance*. New York: Wiley.

**47** Sachdeva, S., Kapoor, P., Tamrakar, A.K., and Noor, R. (2015). Nano-composite dental resins: an overview. *Ann. Dent. Special* 3 (2): 52–55.

**48** Al-Ateeg M.A., Al-Ghamdi A.S., Al-Otaibi M.G., Al-Rasheed K.H., Al-Otaibi A.F., Magdy N.M. Surface gloss of resin composite restorative materials finished/polished with different system. *IOSR-JDMS* 2018; 17(6): 48–53.

**49** Myller, K., Silvennoinen, R., and Peiponen, K.E. (2003). Gloss inspection of metallic products by diffractive optical element based sensor. *Opto-Electron. Rev.* 11 (1): 35–38.

**50** Egilmez, F., Ergun, G., Cekic-Nagas, I. et al. (2012). Estimation of the surface gloss of dental nano composites as a function of color measuring geometry. *Am. J. Dent.* 25 (4): 220–226.

**51** Lu, H., Roeder, L.B., Lei, L., and Powers, J.M. (2005). Effect of surface roughness on stain resistance of dental resin composites. *J. Esthet. Restor. Dent.* 17: 102–108.

**52** Kakaboura, A., Fragouli, M., Rahiotis, C., and Silikas, N. (2007). Evaluation of surface characteristics of dental composites using profilometry, scanning electron, atomic force microscopy and gloss-meter. *J. Mater. Sci. Mater. Med.* 18: 155–163.

**53** Bennett, H.E. and Porteus, J.O. (1961). Relation between surface roughness and specular reflectance at normal incidence. *J. Opt. Soc. Am.* 51: 123–129.

**54** Ferracane, J.L., Condon, J.R., and Mitchem, J.C. (1992). Evaluation of subsurface defects created during the finishing of composites. *J. Dent. Res.* 71: 1628–1632.

**55** Pacifici, E., Bossù, M., Giovannetti, A. et al. (2013). Surface roughness of glass ionomer cements indicated for uncooperative patients according to surface protection treatment. *Ann. Stomatol. (Roma)* 4 (3–4): 250–258.

# 6

# Simulation of Oral Environment

| KEY CONCEPTS |
|---|
| • Knowledge of various methods of simulation of the oral environment to closely match the clinical milieu.<br>• Understanding of the simulation of saliva, temperature variations in the oral cavity, masticatory forces, pH changes, effects of tooth brushing, and periodontium. |

In several in vitro studies, the simulation of oral environment is of prime importance so as to obtain a result that could possibly match the results upon clinical trial and subsequent techno commercial suitability of either a material, technique, or technology. For the laboratory assessment of dental restorative materials, simulation of saliva, temperature change, masticatory forces, pH cycling, tooth brushing, and periodontium is required for the suitable replication of the oral environment.

| Good to Know |
|---|
| Average time taken to brush by a person daily is 120 seconds. Based on this estimation, the maximum contact time for one tooth surface per day is 5 seconds. Thus, if the total brushing time is calculated to be 60 minutes, it is equivalent to 1 year of brushing. |

a) **Saliva:** Saliva is an important component of the oral cavity. Saliva contains calcium, phosphate, and fluoride in a supersaturated state. The saliva also contains a variety of proteins responsible for the lubrication function and for the formation of acquired pellicle, which diminishes the direct contact of acids with the tooth surface. Furthermore, the saliva can act as a diluting agent removing acids gradually by swallowing process. Various therapies are initially tested using in vitro protocols, and saliva is usually used as a control to mimic oral conditions. However, due to the constant contact of saliva with restorative materials in the oral cavity, they may affect the physical, mechanical, and biological integrity of restorative materials. There is no standardization of the

*Manual of Laboratory Testing Methods for Dental Restorative Materials*, First Edition.
Paromita Mazumdar and Deepshikha Chowdhury.

Companion website: www.wiley.com/go/mazumdar/dental-restorative-materials

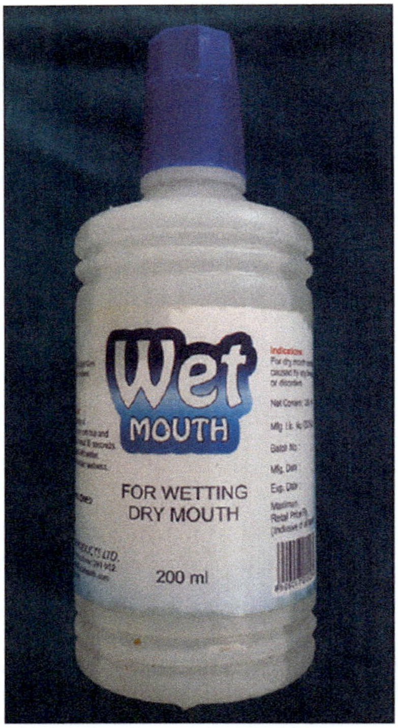


**Figure 6.1** Commercially available artificial saliva.

composition of artificial saliva, and variations in the composition can result in higher or less remineralization. Several compositions are found in different studies which are as follows [1, 2]:

1) Saliva – (0.33 g $KH_2PO_4$, 0.34 g $Na_2HPO_4$, 1.27 g KCl, 0.16 g NaSCN, 0.58 g NaCl, 0.17 g $CaCl_2$, 0.16 g $NH_4Cl$, 0.2 g urea, 0.03 g glucose, 0.002 g ascorbic acid, 2.7 g mucin in 1000 ml distilled water/pH 7);
2) Saliva – (0.1029g $CaCl_2$ _$2H_2O$, 0.040 66 g $MgCl_2$, 0.544 g $KH_2PO_4$, 4.766 g Hepes buffer acid form, 2.2365 g KCl in 1000 ml distilled water/pH 7);
3) Saliva – (0.381 g NaCl, 0.213 g $CaCl_2$ _2H2O, 1.114 g KCl, 0.738 g $KH_2PO_4$, and 2.2 g mucin in 1000 ml distilled water/pH 7);
4) Saliva – (2g methyl-p-hydroxybenzoate, 10 g sodium carboxymethyl cellulose, 0.625 g KCl, 0.059 g $MgCl_2$ _$6H_2O$, 0.166 g $CaCl_2$ _$2H_2O$, 0.804 g $K_2HPO_4$ and 0.326 g $KH_2PO_4$ in 1000 ml of water/pH 7).

Commercially available products such as "Wet Mouth" by ICPA health products, Mumbai, India, "Aquoral" by Esteve Pharmaceuticals, Spain, "Biotene" by Glaxo Smith and Klein, India as artificial saliva (as shown in Figure 6.1).

**Good to Know**

Most of the commercially available artificial saliva contain water, glycerin, carboxymethylcellulose (CMC) and minerals such as calcium, phosphate, and fluoride. The choice of CMC is justifiable to mimic the visco adhesive nature of human saliva.

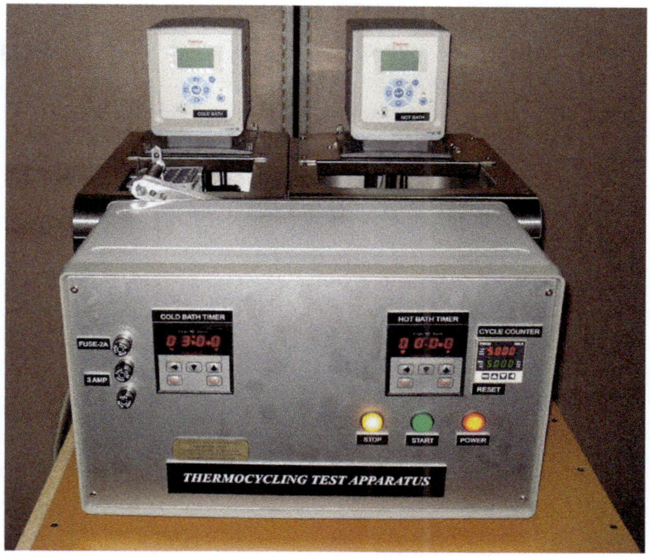


**Figure 6.2** Water bath thermocycling.

b) **Temperature change:** in the oral environment can lead to degradation of dental materials with time. Color change, cracks, fragmentation, and loss of marginal seal may occur. In a study by C.W. Barclay in 2005 studied the intraoral temperature range which was found to vary between 0 and 70 °C [3]. Temperature change can be simulated by thermocycling in deionized water baths (as shown in Figure 6.2) for 15 seconds, at 5–55 ± 2 °C which can be submitted to 500, 1000, 5000,10 000 cycles. In a study by Gale and Darvell et al. [4], 10 000 cycles are equivalent to approximately 1 year of in vivo function. It is also important for the success of restoration to have a value of coefficient of thermal expansion (CTE) as close to that of tooth structure.

| Materials | Coefficient of thermal expansion (ppm/°C) |
|---|---|
| Enamel | 11.8 |
| Dentin | 8.0 |
| Acrylic resin | 90 |
| Porcelain | 4 |
| Amalgam | 25 |
| Composite resin | 25–60 |
| Silicate cements | 10 |

**Good to Know**

The CTE of tooth structure is generally the reference against which the thermal expansion behavior of restorative materials is judged. The mismatch of thermal expansion and contraction between a restoration and the tooth structure may cause stresses to develop at the interface of these two materials, which may have unfavorable effects on the margins and eventually lead to microleakage.

c) **Masticatory forces and their direction:** The teeth and the restorations are subjected to masticatory forces which are a complex set of forces in the form of tensile, shear, compressive, and a combination of these. The average masticatory force for males range from 118 to 142 pounds, while for females, it ranges from 70 to 99 pounds. Masticatory force for anteriors is 29–51 pounds, for premolars is 65 pounds, and for molars, it is 91–198 pounds [5, 6].

A variety of bite force recording devices with different designs and working principles have been used to record bite force, but no single device is capable to record all the required forces.

The bite force devices can either be mechanical or electrical or combination of both. The earlier devices were mechanical inbuilt. Nowadays, sensitive electronic devices are used in most of the bite force devices. Such devices are both accurate and precise enough for common load measuring purposes. Most of the devices can record a wide range of force in Newton (N), (50–800 N) with accuracy (10 N) and precision (80%). These devices use load cells (transducers) to convert force to electrical energy that may be based on one of the following working principles. In humans, bite forces are typically measured using strain gages, pressure-sensitive films, and piezoelectric sensors [7].

## 6.1 Strain gauge Transducers

The strain gauge transducers are devices that consist of a metal plate or fork. On loading, these metal plates undergo deformation, due to which its resistance changes, which, in turn, results in a change in electric potential or voltage. This change in voltage can be calibrated with a known weight to indicate the applied load [8, 9].

## 6.2 Piezoelectric Transducers

When subjected to force, certain crystalline material (e.g. quartz) produces charges on their surface that is directly proportional to the rate of change of that force. These crystals are called as piezoelectric crystals. The produced signals are in the form of a small electric charge and therefore need to be amplified to give a significant reading of load on the material. The whole assembly is called as piezoelectric transducer.

Piezoelectric force transducers using quartz crystals as the active element are readily available commercially. Recently, manufacturing of piezoelectric material in the form of thin foil sheets has been made possible. Using these foils as the active element, an occlusal force transducer can be fabricated that is <2 mm in thickness. It helps to measure occlusal forces with lesser jaw separation than in bite force devices using strain gage transducers. These foils can be cut into any desired shape and size [10].

## 6.3 Pressure Transducers

The pressure transducers consist of a chamber filled with a fluid or air. When subjected to force, the pressure within the chamber increases. This increase in pressure can be transmitted to pressure gage for measurement. Based on the contents of chamber, the pressure transducers can be of two types: pneumatic (air is the medium) and hydraulic (liquid is the medium) [11].

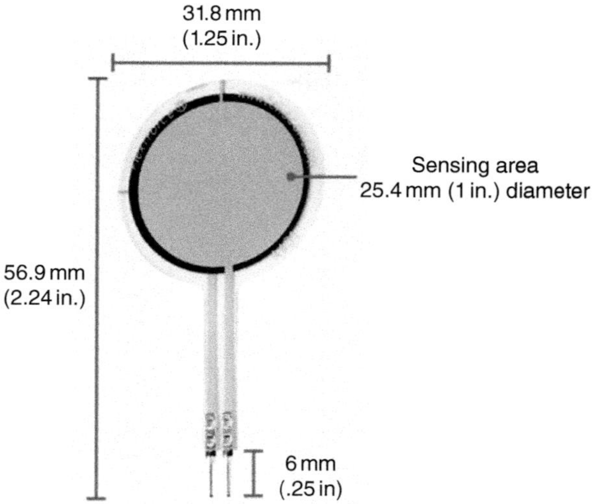


**Figure 6.3** Flexiforce sensor A401.

Some of the commercially available devices for masticatory force measurement include: Dentoforce 2 (ITL AB, Sollentuna, Sweden), IDDK (Kratos, Cotia, São Paulo, Brazil), and T Scan system (Tekscan, Inc., South Boston, MA). These devices have a liquid crystal display (LCD) screen, where a numerical value of the load is displayed.

The Flexiforce sensor A401 (Tekscan Inc., South Boston, USA) (as shown in Figure 6.3) is capable of measuring all types of loads, and thus, it is considered as a strain gage (for measuring sensor flexural loads) and also as a load cell (for measuring vertical loads applied to the sensor). Thus, it can absorb all types of loads applied from the teeth to sensor during mastication and displays interactions quantitatively in Newton (N) using a designed circuit

## 6.4 Cyclic Loading Apparatus

Recently, a cyclic loading apparatus has been designed to simulate the masticatory forces. The Cyclic Loading Apparatus design (as shown in Figure 6.4) was first given by Fruits in 2002. It has been designed to study the effect of flexural strength on the cervical region of the tooth. The force from the bumper is applied to the occlusal half of the clinical crown. With the specimen in a fixed position, the drums are rotated and contact either the buccal or lingual surface of the specimen thus cyclically loading the specimen in the buccal and lingual directions. After load from a particular direction, the specimen recovers under no load and then again the load is applied from an opposite direction. The disc is rotated at 35 rpm and allowed a recovery time of 0.28 seconds between each impact. Each specimen is subjected approximately 8400 cycles and then removed [12].

d) **pH cycling:** An optimal pH of the oral cavity ranges between 6.8 and 7.2. However, changes in pH results in demineralization/remineralization of the dental hard tissues. A pH below 5.5 is known to initiate demineralization of enamel. Acidic pH can reduce

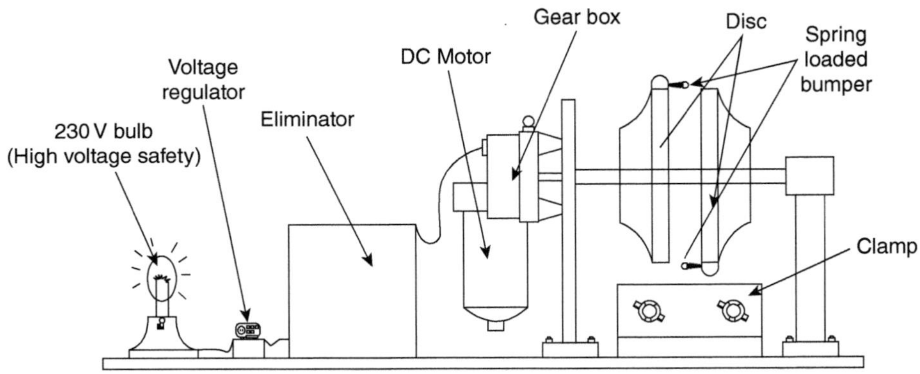


**Figure 6.4** Diagrammatic representation of the cyclic loading apparatus.

the hardness and increase the surface roughness of restorative materials thus reducing the restoration longevity. Also, the increased roughness results in bacterial adherence, plaque accumulation, risk of secondary caries, and alteration of color.

To induce artificial carious lesion or to study demineralization and remineralization of enamel and also to study the effect of pH changes on restorative material, pH cycling is necessary. The oral cavity is subjected to pH change throughout the day. This dynamic process of demineralization and subsequent remineralization alters the properties of tooth as well as the restorative materials.

The composition of the demineralization and remineralization solutions is standardized to obtain a suitable pH to simulate the process [13].

Demineralizing solution (1.4 mM Ca, 0.9 mM P, 0.03 ppm F, 0.05 M acetate buffer, pH 5.0) and Remineralizing solution (1.5 mM Ca, 0.9 mM P, 0.05 ppm F, 0.1 M Tris buffer, pH 7.0) can be used. Immersion time in demineralizing solution can be for 15 minutes or 30 minutes and can extend up to 60 minutes and afterward, immersed for the remaining time in remineralizing solution. The dental materials are also subjected to pH testing (as shown in Figure 6.5).

e) **Tooth brushing**: Brushing effect and the effect of dentifrices on the surface properties of tooth as well as various dental materials are studied very commonly to understand time-dependent behavior of dental restorative materials and also natural tooth substrates during regular daily human practices. Brushing on the specimens manually results in uneven force distribution, strokes as well as difference in the motion. Thus to closely simulate in vivo conditions, customized brushing machines are prepared in order to standardize the in vitro tests. The customized brushing model consisting of a direct current motor, handle, and a wooden base can be constructed. This device is electrically operated (as shown in Figure 6.6). The apparatus has a screw and wedge design that facilitates easy to-and-fro motion of the toothbrush. The samples are placed below the brush head of the automated customized tooth brushing machine. The bristles of the toothbrush are aligned without pressure contacting the specimen surface in perpendicular fashion, and a linear cleaning movement of 3-cm length can be selected for the experiments with manual toothbrush to simulate the most natural brushing method used by patients, which is simple horizontal motion (Scrub Technique).

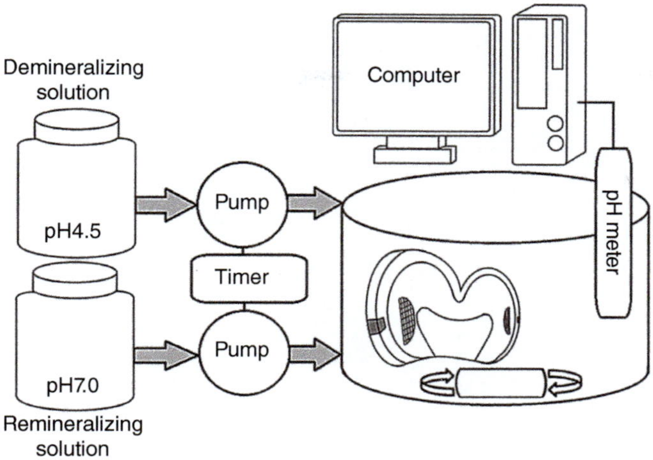


**Figure 6.5** Experimental set-up for pH cycling.

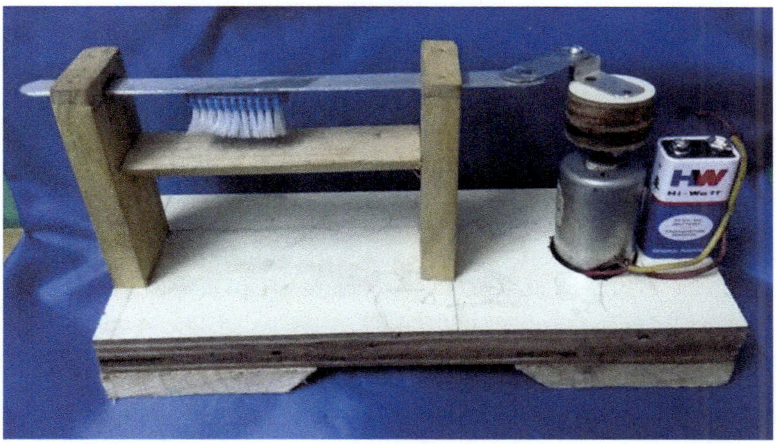

**Figure 6.6** Customized automated tooth brushing machine.

| **Good to Know** |
| --- |
| Slurry of the dentifrice (1 : 3 ratio of water, tooth paste) is prepared according to EN ISO 11609:2010 standard (Dentistry-Toothpastes: Requirements, test methods, and marking). |

A force of 2 N is chosen for brushing. The cleaning force is generated using a compressing spring and an extending screw. Water and toothpaste are mixed in a ratio of 1:3 by weight and spread over the mounted specimens using a measuring scoop before tooth brushing [14].

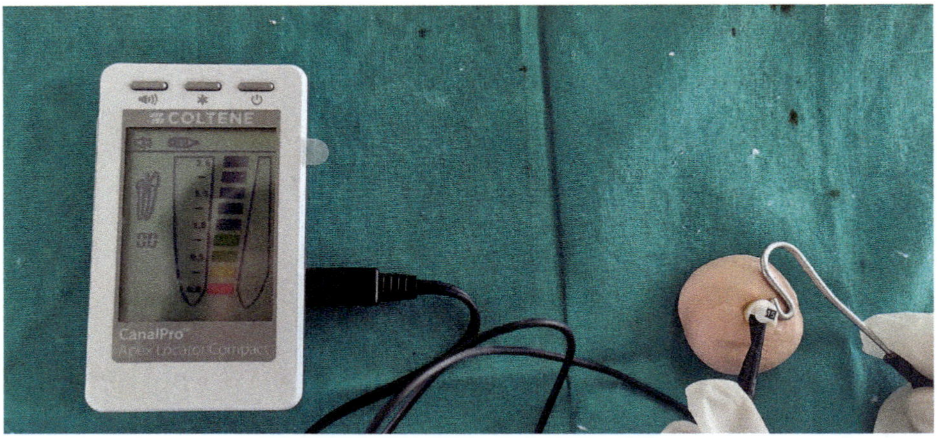


**Figure 6.7** Tooth embedded in alginate to simulate periodontium during in vitro testing of accuracy of electronic apex locator for working length determination.

The brushing time estimation is crucial as it denotes the maximum contact time for one tooth surface per day [15].

f) **Periodontium:** The periodontal ligament is a soft connective tissue which joins the tooth root to the alveolus and provides anchorage to the tooth in the alveolar bone. Its thickness ranges from 0.1 to 0.3 mm. It helps in absorbing occlusal loads and distributes them toward the bone, thereby preventing fracture of the teeth.

The periodontal ligament, if possible, should be reproduced in the laboratory experiment in order to simulate the clinical reality more accurately. A 0.2–0.3 mm thick material should envelope the tooth at the level of cemento enamel junction (CEJ) till below the root apex. Several materials such as alginate, polyether impression material, polyvinyl acetate adhesive, polyvinylsiloxane impression material, cyanoacrylate adhesive, and epoxy resin adhesive have been used in several studies (as shown in Figure 6.7). It is very important that the material must have a non-linear and viscous behavior similar to the periodontium. Due to the similarity of modulus of elasticity of the periodontium and alginate, polyether and polyvinyl siloxane impression materials, they can accurately simulate the periodontium in comparison to the other materials [16].

**Key Points**

1) For in vitro assessment of restorative materials, simulation of saliva, temperature change, masticatory forces, pH cycling, tooth brushing, and periodontium is most commonly done in order to replicate the complex oral environment as closely as possible.
2) Artificial saliva maybe prepared in the laboratory in definite ionic concentrations, or it may be procured commercially. For the commercially available saliva substitutes, the composition must closely match with that of saliva.

3) Temperature change in the oral cavity is simulated by thermocycling the specimens in a water bath within a temperature range of 5–55 °C for the required number of cycles.
4) The oral cavity is subjected to a complex set of forces which are recorded by different bites for recording devices. These devices primarily include strain gages, pressure-sensitive films, and piezoelectric devices.
5) pH cycling is done to replicate the pH changes which take place in the oral cavity that results in remineralization and demineralization. These changes can also alter the properties of the restorative materials.
6) Tooth brushing abrasion primarily leads to changes in surface roughness, microhardness of teeth as well as restorative materials. Manual simulation causes discrepancies in the outcome of the experiment; thus, automated brushing machines are used for this purpose.
7) The periodontium is simulated because the forces of mastication dissipate through the tooth to the periodontium. The materials that are used should have viscoelastic properties similar to that of the periodontium.

## References


**1** Amal, A.S.S, Hussain, S., and Jalaluddin, M. A. (2015).Preparation of artificial saliva formulation. *International Conference ICB Pharma II*, T07, 10–30.

**2** Pytko-Polonczyk, J., Jakubik, A., Przeklasa-Bierowiec, A., and Muszynska, B. (2017). Artificial saliva and its use in biological experiments. *J. Physiol. Pharmacol.* 68: 807–813.

**3** Barclay, C.W., Spence, D., and Laird, W.R.E. (2006). Intra-oral temperatures during function. *J. Oral Rehabil.* 32: 886–894.

**4** Gale, M.S. and Darvell, B.W. (1999). Thermal cycling procedures for laboratory testing of dental restorations. *J. Dent.* 27: 89–99.

**5** Koc, D., Dogan, A., and Bek, B. (2010). Bite force and influential factors on bite force measurements: a literature review. *Eur. J. Dent.* 4 (2): 223–232.

**6** Proffit, W.R., Fields, H.W., and Nixon, W.L. (1983). Occlusal forces in normal-and long-face adults. *J. Dent. Res.* 62 (5): 566–570.

**7** Verma, T.P., Kumathalli, K.I., Jain, V., and Kumar, R. (2017). Bite force recording devices – a review. *J. Clin. Diagn. Res.* 11 (9): ZE01–ZE05.

**8** Lyons, M.F. and Baxendale, R.H. (1990). A preliminary electromyographic study of bite force and jaw-closing muscle fatigue in human subjects with advanced tooth wear. *J. Oral Rehabil.* 17 (4): 311–318.

**9** Bates, J.F., Stafford, G.D., and Harrison, A. (1975). Masticatory function—a review of the literature. *J. Oral Rehabil.* 2 (4): 349–361.

**10** Könönen, M., Klemetti, E., Waltimo, A. et al. (2006). Tooth wear in maxillary anterior teeth from 14 to 23 years of age. *Acta Odontol. Scand.* 64 (1): 55–58.

**11** Lyons, M.F., Cadden, S.W., Baxendale, R.H., and Yemm, R. (1996). Twitch interpolation in the assessment of the maximum force-generating capacity of the jaw-closing muscles in man. *Arch. Oral Biol.* 41 (12): 1161–1168.

**12** Alberto, R.F. and de Ataide, I.D.N. (2007). Effect of cyclical lateral forces on microleakage of cervical resin composite restorations. *J. Conserv. Dent.* 10: 5–13.

**13** Buzalaf, M.A., Hannas, A.R., Magalhães, A.C. et al. (2010). pH-cycling models for in vitro evaluation of the efficacy of fluoridated dentifrices for caries control: strengths and limitations. *J. Appl. Oral Sci.* 18 (4): 316–334.

**14** Mazumdar, P., Chowdhury, D., Chatterjee, S., and Jajoo, N. (2019). Effect of four different dentifrices applied by customized automated brushing device on enamel surface abrasion: an in vitro profilometric study. *J. Conserv. Dent.* 22 (2): 191–195.

**15** Athawale, R., Srinath, S.K., and Chowdary, C. (2018). Comparative evaluation of enamel abrasivity of different commercially available dentifrices – an *in vitro* study. *J. Indian Assoc. Public Health Dent.* 16: 78–82.

**16** Papadogiannis, D., Lakes, R., Palaghias, G., and Papadogiannis, Y. (2011). Effect of storage time on the viscoelastic properties of elastomeric impression materials. *J. Prosthodont. Res.* 56: 11–18.

# 7

# Extra Mile: Biofilm Models and Assessment of Biofilms in Restorative Dentistry

**KEY CONCEPTS**

- Understanding of the oral cavity microflora.
- Ability to differentiate between plaque and biofilm.
- In depth knowledge on biofilms, their virulence factors, formation in the oral cavity.
- Idea about the different in vitro biofilm models and the experimental design.

As we have moved forward in the field of science and art of dentistry, we have begun to realize that the subject is not as mechanical as it was perceived to be. The understanding of the disease processes has evolved over time along with the treatment approaches. It is now known and accepted that many of the dental diseases are bacterial in nature and preventive approaches must be thought of instead of only corrective approaches after a damage has occurred. Though this chapter on biofilm is not directly related to the book title, but an insight into the same will make the manual more complete since there is an increasing interest in developing and testing dental materials for the ability of attracting less biofilm and bacterial adhesion by virtue of improved properties better surface finish. Multispecies oral biofilm developing on the surface of teeth or restorative materials or endodontic materials leads to degradation of the materials altering the structural stability. Oral ecosystem is a dynamic environment inhabited by more than one thousand types of microorganisms.

Bacteria are microscopic, single-celled organisms that thrive in diverse environments. Bacteria (singular: bacterium) are classified as prokaryotes, which are single-celled organisms with a simple internal structure that lacks a nucleus and contains DNA that either floats freely in a twisted, thread-like mass called the nucleoid, or in separate, circular pieces called plasmids. Bacteria grow on solid media as colonies. A colony is defined as a visible mass of microorganisms all originating from a single mother cell; therefore, a colony constitutes a clone of bacteria all genetically alike. The complex environment harbors almost 700 species of microorganism. The main cause of pathogenic process in the oral environment is biofilms. Planktonic bacteria attach themselves reversibly to a surface, form a microcolony, and produce a polymer matrix around the biofilm. They adhere to both tissue surfaces and artificial surfaces such as restorative materials and prosthesis

*Manual of Laboratory Testing Methods for Dental Restorative Materials*, First Edition.
Paromita Mazumdar and Deepshikha Chowdhury.

Companion website: www.wiley.com/go/mazumdar/dental-restorative-materials

ultimately leading to dental decay. It also reduces the lifespan of the dental materials and limits their clinical performance. The restorative materials that have superior ability to inhibit bacterial adhesion, biofilm formation, and thereby reducing the chances of failure are beneficial to the patient. Clinicians need to choose restorative materials by analyzing properties and qualities, and experimental research in the same direction will be useful in selection process. Oral biofilms can further affect the tissues surrounding the tooth where they cause inflammatory processes of the gingiva, and when persistent, damage to the alveolar process can, in the worst case, result in tooth loss [1]. Biofilms are conglomerates of microorganisms (bacteria, algae, and fungi) that adhere to biological and nonbiological surfaces and are functionally organized in layers [2]. For biofilm formation, microorganisms generally require a humid environment to resist dehydration [3]. Microorganisms organize into biofilms to protect against external stress in a specific environment [4, 5]. In addition to mechanical stability, biofilm formation stimulates synergistic interactions, ensures survival in periods of starvation, and prevents the displacement of extracellular enzymes.

Biofilm is a mode of microbial growth where dynamic communities of interacting sessile cells are irreversibly attached to a solid substratum, as well as to each other, and are embedded in a matrix of extracellular polymeric substances (EPS).

## 7.1 Difference Between Dental Plaque and Biofilm

Dental plaque is a structurally and functionally organized biofilm. Plaque forms in an ordered way and has a diverse microbial composition that, in health, remains relatively stable over time (microbial homeostasis). Biofilms are less susceptible to antimicrobial agents, while microbial communities can display enhanced pathogenicity (pathogenic synergism). The structure of the plaque biofilm might restrict the penetration of antimicrobial agents, while bacteria growing on a surface grow slowly and display a novel phenotype, one consequence of which is a reduced sensitivity to inhibitors. Plaque is natural and contributes (like the resident microflora of all other sites in the body) to the normal development of the physiology and defenses of the host.

## 7.2 Virulence Factors of Biofilms

**There are several factors that contribute to the antimicrobial resistance in bacterial biofilms such as**:

1) types of resident bacterial species,
2) nature of bacterial adherence to substrate,
3) physico-chemical characteristics of the substrate,
4) thickness of the biofilm,
5) bacterial cell density,
6) amount of EPS, and
7) phenotypical/genotypical modification of the resident bacteria [6, 7]

Typically, different antimicrobial resistance mechanisms may act concurrently or synergistically in a biofilm structure, and understanding some of these mechanisms is the key to developing biofilm model systems for experimental research in restorative dentistry [7].

## 7.3 Biofilm Formation

During the development of a biofilm, the resident bacterial cells proliferate, leading to expansion of the biofilm structure. In this stage, the monolayer of microbes (primary colonizers) attracts the secondary colonizers, forming microcolonies, and the collection of microcolonies gives rise to the final structure of the biofilm.

Ultrastructurally, a biofilm consists of a population of bacterial cells attached irreversibly to a substrate and encased in a hydrated, polyanionic matrix of EPS, proteins, polysaccharides, and nucleic acids.

## 7.4 Microorganisms in Oral Biofilms

Pioneer colonizers in oral biofilms have been identified as *Streptococcus sanguinis, Streptococcus oralis, Streptococcus gordonii, Streptococcus mitis, Streptococcus mutans, Streptococcus sobrinus, Actinomyces naeslundii*, and *Capnocytophaga ochracea* [8].

After pioneer colonizers, secondary colonizers, consisting of various species depending on the bacterial composition of the environment, follow; these species can be used to predict the bacterial composition of the mature biofilm [8].

The mature stage of the oral biofilm usually occurs after three to five days and is characterized by thickness and microbial composition. Mature biofilms have high microbiological variability and contain mainly rods that are absent in growing biofilms. The main bacteria in the mature biofilms on most materials are identified as *S. oralis* [9, 10].

## 7.5 In vitro Biofilm Models

According to International Union of Pure and Applied Chemistry (IUPAC), biofilm is a three-dimensional structure in which an aggregate of microorganisms is embedded in a self-produced matrix of extra polymeric substances adhering to each other and/or to surface. In the oral cavity, biofilms may be found on dental hard and soft tissues and surfaces of restorations. Formation of biofilm involves the steps of pellicle formation, bacterial colonization, and biofilm maturation. Bacterial adhesion is a microbial accumulation on different surfaces. Human dental plaque is a complex biofilm that is present on tooth as well as restorative materials. In the oral cavity, biofilm may be found on dental hard and soft tissues, associated with caries and periodontal diseases and on restorative materials. Biofilm consists of EPS 80% and microcolonies 20%. Several reports suggest that restorative materials may have anti-bacterial activity or may even induce the growth of bacteria.

Certain restorative composite resins may have properties that make them more susceptible to biofilm formation leading to secondary care and even periodontitis. Various in vivo and in vitro studies have demonstrated that oral bacteria attachment and biofilm formation occur at a higher frequency on dental restorative materials than on natural teeth in the oral cavity. Biological interaction of microorganisms with dental materials plays a crucial role in determining the successful function of these materials. Hence, bacterial adhesion and biofilm analysis is assuming importance nowadays.

Bacterial biofilms are developed in order to study the microbial interactions between bacteria and host immune cells. Currently, they are more commonly grown to test the antimicrobial efficacy of different restorative materials. Laboratory models are conventionally used to mimic natural biofilms for different experimental purposes.

These in vitro biofilms are easy to control and useful in obtaining standardized biofilm models with predictable structure and behavior. There are two types of biofilm models, static and dynamic.

The static biofilm models use different substrates (e.g. glass, polycarbonate, silicon, hydroxyl apatite, nitrocellulose, enamel, dentin) to grow biofilms, while the dynamic biofilm models use reactor or fermenting systems to grow biofilms on a particular substrate. Both aerobic and anaerobic environments can be employed for in vitro biofilm development [6–8].

### 7.5.1 Static Biofilm Models

The static biofilm system generates biofilms that have exhausted important nutrient components at the end of an overnight incubation. In this system, a number of biofilms can be handled at any given time and it does not require time-consuming sterilization and set-up procedures, allowing it to be used as automated equipment to rapidly test thousands to millions of samples for biological activity at molecular level. This system provides a basis for the rapid screening of biofilm mutants, biomass development, and biofilm-forming capacity, as well as extracellular matrix (ECM) composition. Essentially, detection of any microbial phenotype that can be easily processed by a microtiter reader can be used for the approach. However, the major limitation of this system is it's incompatibility with a confocal laser scanning microscope which is usually preferred for studying biofilms [11–13].

### 7.5.2 Dynamic Biofilm Models

The biofilms that experience a continuous flow of medium supplemented with fresh nutrients are dynamic biofilm models. The flow cell system is one of the most utilized dynamic models. It consists of a transparent chamber of fixed depth through which the growth medium flows. The inlet tubing supplies growth medium, and the outlet tubing drains the medium to a waste reservoir. The growth medium is passed through the cell with the aid of a peristaltic pump, which controls the flow rate of the medium. Pre-fabricated flow cell systems are available commercially, or they can be custom-made based on any particular application. In conjunction with a microscope, charge-coupled-device (CCD) camera, or confocal laser scanning microscopy (CLSM), this method can be used to observe the early events in biofilm formation in real time [11].

Chemostats are also used to grow dynamic biofilms of microbes on experimental substrates submerged within the chemostat. One of the most important features of chemostats is that microbial biofilms can be grown at a constant rate and under constant culture conditions (temperature, pH) [7].

Similar to chemostat, there is another category of reactors in which biofilms are formed on thin filter membranes in a physiological steady state. These systems permit evaluation of growth rate dependence and cell-cycle specificity of antibacterial agents.

Finally, there are constant depth reactors in which surface growth is periodically removed to maintain a constant geometry of the biofilm. In these reactors, microorganisms can be grown in a physiological steady state with all culture parameters constant. The system can generate large numbers of biofilms with comparable and reproducible data [6, 7, 11, 14].

## 7.6 Applications of In vitro Biofilm Models

**These in vitro bacterial biofilm models are routinely applied to**:

i) examine the adherence of specific bacterial species to any biomaterial surface
ii) study the nature and pattern of early microbial biofilm formation on a particular substrate
iii) study the interaction between different biofilm bacteria and host immune cells and
iv) test the efficacy of antimicrobial agents or antimicrobial treatment strategies [15, 16].

## 7.7 Factors Affecting Biofilm Adhesion to Restorative Materials

Generally, the negatively charged bacterial cell membrane is more prone to adhere to positively charged surfaces than to negatively charged or uncharged surfaces; hence, surface charge has a sizeable influence on biofilm formation. Furthermore, biofilm formation is dependent on surface energy. Bacterial adhesion is more potent on hydrophilic surfaces than on hydrophobic surfaces. Finally, the roughness and topography of a surface influence the extent of bacterial adhesion on the material surface. Hence, all these factors influence the rate of biofilm formation [17–19].

## 7.8 Sample Preparation for Biofilm Study on Restorative Materials

Apart from the in vitro biofilm models, natural oral biofilm has always been an area of interest for researchers. If biofilm has to be studied clinically, the sample has to be designed in a manner so that the restorative material is in constant touch with the oral environment. Ex vivo studies have been done which include placing a disc of restorative material attached to an acrylic plate or a bite splint which the participant has to wear for a designated time period. The restorative material blocks are then assessed in a laboratory using the methods described in Chapter 3.

## 7.9 Use of Biofilm Assays

**Biofilm assays are used to characterize factors such as:**

i) number and phenotype of the microorganism,
ii) dead/living cells in the population
iii) state of maturation
iv) thickness (mono-layered or multilayered),
v) structure (homogeneous, irregular, dense, porous),
vi) surface topography (peaks and valleys) of biofilms.

**Different techniques such as:**

i) microbiological culture techniques,
ii) colorimetric techniques,
iii) microscopic techniques,
iv) physical methods, thickness, weight, area, and density measurements
v) biochemical methods: biomass and ECM
vi) molecular methods are applied to biofilm assays.

## 7.10 Biofilm Formation on Restorative Materials

There are several restorative materials which are routinely used in the oral cavity. It has been seen that gold casting alloy, base metal alloy, dental amalgam, and glazed porcelain have the least amount of biofilm formation on their surface. Dental amalgam and gold casting alloy are metallic materials with high electrical conductivity that plays a role in bacterial adhesion. This is because bacteria are negatively charged and attracted to positively charged conducting metallic materials. However, the biofilm formed on these materials have low viability thus explaining the clinical longevity of these materials. Resin composite and glass ionomer have shown greater amount of biofilm formation which may be attributed to the hydrophilicity of glass ionomer and surface roughness and wear of resin composites [20, 21].

**Key Points**

1) Biofilm is a mode of microbial growth where dynamic communities of interacting sessile cells are irreversibly attached to a solid substratum, as well as to each other, and are embedded in a matrix of extracellular polymeric substances (EPS).
2) Dental plaque is a biofilm that is more structurally and functionally organized.
3) The different virulence factors of biofilm makes them resistant to antibiotics.
4) There are two types of biofilm models that are used for in vitro studies – static and dynamic.

## References


1 Papapanou, P.N., Mariano, S., Nurcan, B. et al. (2018). Periodontitis: consensus report of workgroup 2 of the 2017 world workshop on the classification of periodontal and Peri-implant diseases and conditions. *J. Periodontol.* 89 (Suppl 1): S173–S182.

2 Marsh, P.D. (2005). Dental plaque: biological significance of a biofilm and community life-style. *J. Clin. Periodontol.* 32 (Suppl 6): 7–15.

3 Bassler, B.L. and Losick, R. (2006). Bacterially speaking. *Cell* 125 (2): 237–246.

4 Chia, N., Woese, C.R., and Goldenfeld, N. (2008). A collective mechanism for phase variation in biofilms. *Proc. Natl. Acad. Sci. U. S. A.* 105 (38): 14597–14602.

5 Shemesh, M., Tam, A., and Steinberg, D. (2007). Differential gene expression profiling of Streptococcus mutans cultured under biofilm and planktonic conditions. *Microbiology* 153 (Pt 5): 1307–1317.

6 Casadevall, A. and Pirofski, L.A. (1999). Host–pathogen interactions: redefining the basic concepts of virulence and pathogenicity. *Infect. Immun.* 67: 3703–3713.

7 Chavez de Paz, L.E. (2007). Redefining the persistent infection in root canals: possible role of biofilm communities. *J. Endod.* 33: 652–662.

8 Souza, J.C., Mota, R.R., Sordi, M.B. et al. (2016). Biofilm formation on different materials used in oral rehabilitation. *Braz. Dent. J.* 27 (2): 141–147.

9 Nobbs, A.H., Lamont, R.J., and Jenkinson, H.F. (2009). Streptococcus adherence and colonization. *Microbiol. Mol. Biol. Rev.* 73 (3): 407–450.

10 Teughels, W., Van Assche, N., Sliepen, I. et al. (2006). Effect of material characteristics and/or surface topography on biofilm development. *Clin. Oral Implants Res.* 17 (Suppl 2): 68–81.

11 Kulasekara, H.D., Ventre, I., Kulasekara, B.R. et al. (2005). A novel two-component system controls the expression of Pseudomonas aeruginosa fimbrial cup genes. *Mol. Microbiol.* 55: 368–380.

12 Watnick, P.I. and Kolter, R. (1999). Steps in the development of a Vibrio cholerae El Tor biofilm. *Mol. Microbiol.* 34: 586–595.

13 Friedman, L. and Kolter, R. (2004). Genes involved in matrix formation in Pseudomonas aeruginosa PA14 biofilms. *Mol. Microbiol.* 51: 675–690.

14 Pavarina, A.C., Dovigo, L.N., Sanitá, P.V. et al. (2011). Dynamic models for in vitro biofilm formation. In: *Biofilms: Formation, Development and Properties* (ed. W.C. Bailey), 125–162. Hauppauge, NY: Nova Science Publishers, Inc.

15 Kishen, A., Sum, C.P., Mathew, S., and Lim, C.T. (2008). Influence of irrigation regimens on the adherence of *Enterococcus faecalis* to root canal dentin. *J. Endod.* 34: 850–854.

16 Mathew, S., Yaw-Chyn, L., and Kishen, A. (2010). Immunogenic potential of *Enterococcus faecalis* biofilm under simulated growth conditions. *J. Endod.* 36: 832–836.

17 Mohr, M., Tosun, S., Arnold, W.H. et al. (2015). Quantification of cell fusion events human breast cancer cells and breast epithelial cells using a Cre-LoxP-based double fluorescence reporter system. *Cell. Mol. Life Sci.* 72 (19): 3769–3782.

18 Song, F., Koo, H., and Ren, D. (2015). Effects of material properties on bacterial adhesion and biofilm formation. *J. Dent. Res.* 94 (8): 1027–1034.

**19** Hannig, C., Helbig, R., Hilsenbeck, J. et al. (2018). Impact of the springtail's cuticle nanotopography on bioadhesion and biofilm formation in vitro and in the oral cavity. *R. Soc. Open Sci.* 5 (7): 171742.

**20** Deng, S. (2019). Biofilm formation and contact angles on dental restorative biomaterials. *Decisions Dentistry* 5 (8): 12–16.

**21** Dekaboruah, E., Suryavanshi, M., and Chettri, D. (2020). Human microbiome: an academic update on human body site specific surveillance and its possible role. *Arch. Microbiol.* 202: 2147–2167.

# Index



*Manual of Laboratory Testing Methods for Dental Restorative Materials*, First Edition.
Paromita Mazumdar and Deepshikha Chowdhury.

Companion website: www.wiley.com/go/mazumdar/dental-restorative-materials